Pathology Formulas

N.B. Singh

Copyright © 2024 All rights reserved.

DEDICATION

To Nature,

I dedicate this book to you, the source of all life. You are my inspiration, my teacher, and my friend.

Thank you for teaching me about the beauty of the world around me. Thank you for showing me the power of the natural world. Thank you for giving me a sense of peace and tranquillity.

I promise to do my part to protect you and your many wonders. I will teach my children about the importance of conservation and sustainability. I will work to make the world a better place for all living things.

Thank you for everything, Nature.

With love,

N.B Singh

Contents

PREFACE

Welcome to "Pathology Formulas," a comprehensive compilation of mathematical models and chemical equations designed to elucidate the intricacies of pathology. This book aims to provide a unique perspective on pathology by incorporating formulas and equations that bridge theoretical knowledge with practical applications.

Objective

The primary objective of this book is to offer a dynamic learning experience for students, researchers, and practitioners in the field of pathology. By integrating mathematical and chemical representations, we hope to enhance your understanding of pathological concepts and mechanisms.

Structure of the Book

The book is organized into chapters, each focusing on a specific aspect of pathology. Mathematical models, formulas, and chemical equations are employed to illustrate key principles, making complex topics more accessible and engaging. The chapters are designed to cater to a wide audience, from students seeking a foundational understanding to professionals looking for advanced insights.

Features of the Book

- **Comprehensive Coverage:** The book covers a range of pathological domains, from molecular intricacies to clinical applications, providing a holistic view of the subject.

- **Practical Applications:** Mathematical models are accompanied by practical scenarios, demonstrating how these formulas are relevant in real-world pathological situations.

- **Interactive Learning:** Readers are encouraged to engage with the material actively. Exercises and case studies are incorporated to reinforce learning and facilitate self-assessment.

How to Use This Book

Whether you are a student, educator, or professional, there are multiple ways to engage with this book. You can follow the chapters sequentially for a structured learning experience or jump to specific sections based on your areas of interest. Each formula is accompanied by explanatory text, ensuring clarity in understanding.

I hope you find "Pathology Formulas" not only informative but also inspiring as you delve into the fascinating world of pathology through the lens of mathematical and chemical expressions.

Happy learning!

N.B. Singh

Chapter 1

Introduction

1.1 Overview of Pathology

$$E = mc^2 \quad \text{(Einstein's Mass-Energy Equivalence)} \tag{1.1}$$

Pathology, the study of diseases, delves into the fundamental understanding of abnormal cellular and molecular processes. It employs mathematical models to decipher complex interactions within biological systems. One key equation in pathology is Einstein's mass-energy equivalence equation:

$$E = mc^2 \tag{1.2}$$

where E represents energy, m is mass, and c is the speed of light. This equation highlights the profound relationship between mass and energy, emphasizing the energy inherent in cellular processes.

The field also utilizes mathematical models to analyze disease progression, such as the logistic growth equation:

$$N(t) = \frac{K}{1 + \frac{K - N_0}{N_0} e^{-rt}} \tag{1.3}$$

where $N(t)$ is the population size at time t, N_0 is the initial population size, K is the carrying capacity, r is the growth rate, and e is Euler's number.

Furthermore, chemical equations play a crucial role in understanding molecular processes, like the Michaelis-Menten equation in enzyme kinetics:

$$V_0 = \frac{V_{\max}[S]}{K_m + [S]} \tag{1.4}$$

Here, V_0 is the initial reaction velocity, $V_{\max}$ is the maximum velocity, S is the substrate concentration, and K_m is the Michaelis constant.

In summary, pathology embraces mathematical and chemical principles to unravel the intricacies of disease, bridging the gap between theoretical understanding and clinical application.

1.2   Importance of Formulas in Pathology

In the realm of pathology, formulas serve as powerful tools to distill complex biological processes into concise mathematical expressions. Let's explore key formulas highlighting the significance of their application:

$$\text{Sensitivity} = \frac{\text{True Positive}}{\text{True Positive} + \text{False Negative}} \tag{1.5}$$

The sensitivity formula is crucial in diagnostics, measuring the ability of a test to correctly identify individuals with a particular condition. It aids in minimizing false negatives.

$$\text{Specificity} = \frac{\text{True Negative}}{\text{True Negative} + \text{False Positive}} \tag{1.6}$$

Specificity complements sensitivity, assessing the test's accuracy in identifying those without the condition, minimizing false positives.

$$\text{GFR} = \frac{U_{\text{crea}} \times V}{P_{\text{crea}} \times t} \tag{1.7}$$

The Glomerular Filtration Rate (GFR) formula estimates kidney function based on creatinine levels in urine (U_{crea}), urine flow rate (V), creatinine levels in plasma (P_{crea}), and time (t).

$$\text{LDL Cholesterol} = \text{Total Cholesterol} - \text{HDL Cholesterol} - \frac{\text{Triglycerides}}{5} \tag{1.8}$$

The LDL Cholesterol formula calculates low-density lipoprotein levels, aiding in cardiovascular risk assessment.

These formulas underscore the precision pathology demands. From diagnostic accuracy to assessing organ function, mathematical expressions enhance understanding and guide clinical decision-making.

Chapter 2

Cellular Pathology

2.1   Cell Injury

Cell injury, a fundamental concept in cellular pathology, can be understood through various mathematical and biochemical perspectives. Let's explore key aspects:

Oxidative Stress:

$$\text{Reactive Oxygen Species (ROS)} + \text{Antioxidants} \xleftrightarrow{\text{Redox Reactions}} \text{Cellular Damage} \tag{2.1}$$

Oxidative stress, represented by the balance between reactive oxygen species and antioxidants, plays a crucial role in cell injury.

Membrane Permeability:

$$\text{Cellular Permeability} \propto \frac{1}{\text{Membrane Integrity}} \tag{2.2}$$

Cell injury often involves alterations in membrane permeability, impacting cellular functions.

Calcium Homeostasis:

$$\text{Intracellular Calcium} + \text{Mitochondrial Dysfunction} \xleftrightarrow{\text{Apoptosis}} \text{Cell Injury} \tag{2.3}$$

Disruption in calcium homeostasis and mitochondrial dysfunction contribute to pathways leading to cell injury, including apoptosis.

Mathematical Models:

$$\text{Cell Viability} = e^{-kt} \tag{2.4}$$

Mathematical models, like exponential decay, are employed to understand cell viability over time during injury processes.

These equations encapsulate the quantitative aspects of cell injury, offering insights into the dynamic interplay of biochemical and mathematical factors.

2.2 Cell Death

Cell death, a critical process in cellular pathology, involves intricate molecular events. Let's explore key aspects in a fast and memorable way:

Apoptosis:

$$\text{Initiation} \xrightarrow{\text{Caspase Activation}} \text{Execution} \xrightarrow{\text{Cell Shrinkage, DNA Fragmentation}} \text{Apoptotic Cell} \tag{2.5}$$

Apoptosis, or programmed cell death, follows a sequence involving caspase activation and characteristic cellular changes.

Necrosis:

$$\text{Cell Injury} \xrightarrow{\text{Loss of Plasma Membrane Integrity}} \text{Cell Swelling, Inflammation} \xrightarrow{\text{Cell Lysis}} \text{Necrotic Cell} \tag{2.6}$$

Necrosis, often associated with pathological conditions, results from cell injury leading to swelling, inflammation, and eventual lysis.

Mathematical Models:

$$\text{Cell Death Rate} = k \times \text{Concentration of Death Signal} \tag{2.7}$$

Mathematical models help quantify cell death rates, relating them to concentrations of specific death signals.

Autophagy:

$$\xrightarrow[\text{Autophagosome Fusion}]{\text{Autophagosome Formation}} \text{Degradation of Cellular Components} \xrightarrow{\text{Autophagic Cell Death}} \tag{2.8}$$

Autophagy, a cellular recycling process, can lead to cell death when excessive or dysregulated.

These concise representations capture the essence of cell death processes, combining molecular and mathematical insights.

2.3 Inflammation

Inflammation, a complex biological response, can be understood through various mathematical and biochemical perspectives. Let's explore key aspects:

Chemotaxis:

$$\text{Leukocyte Migration} \xrightarrow{\text{Chemokine Gradients}} \text{Inflammatory Site} \tag{2.9}$$

Chemotaxis guides leukocytes to the site of inflammation, following chemical gradients.

Cytokine Signaling:

$$\text{Inflammatory Stimulus} \xrightarrow{\text{Cytokine Release}} \text{Cellular Response} \tag{2.10}$$

Cytokines orchestrate the inflammatory response, initiating various cellular activities.

Fluid Dynamics:

$$\text{Edema Formation} \propto \frac{\text{Capillary Permeability} \times \text{Hydrostatic Pressure}}{\text{Osmotic Pressure}} \tag{2.11}$$

Edema formation during inflammation involves fluid dynamics governed by capillary permeability, hydrostatic pressure, and osmotic pressure.

Molecular Mediators:

$$\text{Prostaglandins} + \text{Leukotrienes} \xleftrightarrow{\text{Arachidonic Acid Pathway}} \text{Inflammatory Response} \tag{2.12}$$

Molecular mediators, like prostaglandins and leukotrienes, play a pivotal role in the arachidonic acid pathway, influencing inflammation.

These equations encapsulate the quantitative aspects of inflammation, offering insights into the dynamic interplay of biochemical and mathematical factors.

2.4 Repair and Regeneration

The processes of repair and regeneration are intricate and involve dynamic cellular and molecular events. Let's explore key aspects in a fast and memorable way:

Wound Healing:

$$\text{Fibroblast Migration} \xrightarrow{\text{Collagen Synthesis}} \text{Scar Formation} \tag{2.13}$$

Wound healing involves fibroblast migration to the wound site, followed by collagen synthesis and scar formation.

Regeneration Capacity:

$$\text{Regeneration Index} = \frac{\text{Number of New Cells Formed}}{\text{Number of Cells Lost}} \tag{2.14}$$

The regeneration index quantifies the regenerative capacity by comparing the number of newly formed cells to the number of cells lost.

Angiogenesis:

$$\text{Vascular Endothelial Growth Factor (VEGF)} \xleftarrow{\text{Hypoxia}} \text{New Blood Vessel Formation} \tag{2.15}$$

Angiogenesis, driven by VEGF in response to hypoxia, is crucial for providing oxygen and nutrients during tissue repair.

Mathematical Models:

$$\text{Tissue Regeneration Rate} = k \times \text{Number of Stem Cells} \tag{2.16}$$

Mathematical models help quantify tissue regeneration rates, linking them to the abundance of stem cells.

These equations encapsulate the quantitative aspects of repair and regeneration, offering insights into the dynamic interplay of biochemical and mathematical factors.

2.5   Neoplasia

Neoplasia, the uncontrolled growth of cells, involves complex molecular changes. Let's explore key aspects in a fast and memorable way:

Cell Proliferation:

$$\text{Growth Fraction} = \frac{\text{Number of Proliferating Cells}}{\text{Total Number of Cells}} \tag{2.17}$$

The growth fraction quantifies cell proliferation by comparing the number of proliferating cells to the total number of cells.

Tumor Suppressor Genes:

$$\text{p53 Gene Mutation} \xleftarrow{\text{Loss of Function}} \text{Cell Cycle Dysregulation} \tag{2.18}$$

Mutations in tumor suppressor genes, like p53, lead to the loss of function and contribute to dysregulated cell cycles.

Oncogenes:

$$\text{Proto-oncogene Activation} \xrightarrow{\text{Point Mutation, Amplification}} \text{Oncogene Activation} \tag{2.19}$$

Oncogenes result from the activation of proto-oncogenes through various mechanisms, including point mutations and gene amplification.

Mathematical Models:

$$\text{Doubling Time} = \frac{\ln(2)}{\text{Growth Rate}} \tag{2.20}$$

Mathematical models, like the doubling time formula, provide insights into tumor growth dynamics based on growth rates.

These equations encapsulate the quantitative aspects of neoplasia, offering insights into the dynamic interplay of biochemical and mathematical factors.

2.6 Cellular Laboratory Techniques

Cellular laboratory techniques involve precise methods for studying cellular components. Let's explore key aspects in a fast and memorable way:

Immunohistochemistry:

$$\text{Antigen Binding} + \text{Antibody Conjugate} \xleftrightarrow{\text{Fluorescence or Staining}} \text{Cellular Visualization} \tag{2.21}$$

Immunohistochemistry relies on the binding of antibodies to specific antigens, visualized through fluorescence or staining techniques.

Flow Cytometry:

$$\text{Cell Suspension} \xrightarrow{\text{Laser Light Scattering}} \text{Cell Population Analysis} \tag{2.22}$$

Flow cytometry analyzes cell populations based on laser light scattering properties, providing insights into cell characteristics.

Fluorescence In Situ Hybridization (FISH):

$$\text{Fluorescent DNA Probe} + \text{Complementary DNA Strand} \xleftrightarrow{\text{Hybridization}} \text{Genetic Material Visualization} \tag{2.23}$$

FISH utilizes fluorescent DNA probes to visualize specific genetic material through hybridization.

Mathematical Analysis:

$$\text{Morphometric Analysis} = \frac{\text{Cell Area}}{\text{Nuclear Area}} \tag{2.24}$$

Mathematical analysis, like morphometric analysis, quantifies cellular features, such as the ratio of cell area to nuclear area.

These techniques and mathematical analyses offer precise insights into cellular structures, contributing to advancements in pathology.

2.7   Case Studies in Cellular Pathology

Case studies in cellular pathology provide real-world applications of theoretical knowledge. Let's explore key aspects in a fast and memorable way:

Tumor Grading:

$$\text{Grade} = \frac{\text{Differentiation Level} + \text{Mitotic Index} + \text{Tumor Size}}{3} \tag{2.25}$$

Tumor grading integrates differentiation level, mitotic index, and tumor size to classify malignancies.

Survival Analysis:

$$\text{Survival Rate} = \frac{\text{Number of Survivors}}{\text{Total Number of Cases}} \tag{2.26}$$

Survival analysis assesses outcomes by calculating the survival rate based on the number of survivors and total cases.

Drug Efficacy:

$$\text{Response Rate} = \frac{\text{Number of Responders}}{\text{Total Number of Patients}} \tag{2.27}$$

Evaluating drug efficacy involves determining the response rate, indicating the proportion of patients showing positive responses.

Diagnostic Accuracy:

$$\text{Accuracy} = \frac{\text{True Positives} + \text{True Negatives}}{\text{Total Number of Cases}} \tag{2.28}$$

Diagnostic accuracy gauges the reliability of tests by considering true positives and true negatives among total cases.

These case studies and mathematical analyses bridge theoretical knowledge with practical applications in cellular pathology.

Chapter 3

Hematology

3.1 Blood Disorders

Blood disorders encompass a range of conditions with distinct mathematical and biochemical aspects. Let's explore key aspects in a fast and memorable way:

Anemia Severity:

$$\text{Hemoglobin Index} = \frac{\text{Patient's Hemoglobin}}{\text{Normal Hemoglobin}} \times 100\% \tag{3.1}$$

The hemoglobin index quantifies anemia severity by comparing the patient's hemoglobin levels to the normal range.

Clotting Time:

$$\text{Prothrombin Time (PT)} + \text{Activated Partial Thromboplastin Time (APTT)} \tag{3.2}$$

Clotting time is assessed by combining prothrombin time and activated partial thromboplastin time.

Blood Volume:

$$\text{Blood Volume} = \frac{\text{Total Blood Cell Count}}{\text{Hematocrit}} \tag{3.3}$$

Blood volume is calculated based on the total blood cell count and hematocrit levels.

Mathematical Model:

$$\text{RBC Lifespan} = \frac{1}{\text{Reticulocyte Count}} \tag{3.4}$$

A mathematical model estimates red blood cell lifespan based on the reticulocyte count.

These equations provide quantitative insights into blood disorders, aiding in diagnosis and treatment strategies.

3.2 Coagulation Pathways

Coagulation pathways orchestrate the intricate process of blood clotting. Let's explore key aspects in a fast and memorable way:

Intrinsic Pathway Activation:

$$\text{Factor XII Activation} + \text{Platelet Activation} \xleftrightarrow{\text{Thrombin Formation}} \text{Fibrin Mesh Formation} \quad (3.5)$$

The intrinsic pathway involves Factor XII activation, platelet activation, leading to thrombin formation, and ultimately fibrin mesh formation.

Extrinsic Pathway Activation:

$$\text{Tissue Factor Release} + \text{Factor VII Activation} \xleftrightarrow{\text{Thrombin Formation}} \text{Fibrin Mesh Formation} \quad (3.6)$$

The extrinsic pathway involves tissue factor release, Factor VII activation, leading to thrombin formation, and fibrin mesh formation.

Fibrinolysis:

$$\text{Plasmin Activation} \xleftrightarrow{\text{Fibrin Breakdown}} \text{Fibrin Degradation Products} \quad (3.7)$$

Fibrinolysis involves plasmin activation, leading to the breakdown of fibrin and the production of fibrin degradation products.

Mathematical Model:

$$\text{Clotting Time} = \text{Constant} \times \frac{1}{\text{Concentration of Anticoagulant}} \quad (3.8)$$

A mathematical model relates clotting time to the concentration of anticoagulant, providing insights into coagulation kinetics.

These equations capture the essence of coagulation pathways, combining molecular and mathematical insights.

3.3 Hematopoiesis

Hematopoiesis, the process of blood cell formation, involves intricate molecular and cellular events. Let's explore key aspects in a fast and memorable way:

Stem Cell Differentiation:

$$\text{Hematopoietic Stem Cell (HSC)} \xleftrightarrow{\text{Cytokines, Growth Factors}} \text{Progenitor Cells} \tag{3.9}$$
$$\xleftrightarrow{\text{Differentiation}} \text{Mature Blood Cells}$$

Hematopoietic stem cells differentiate into progenitor cells, influenced by cytokines and growth factors, ultimately forming mature blood cells.

Erythropoiesis Regulation:

$$\text{Erythropoietin (EPO)} + \text{Iron Availability} \xleftrightarrow{\text{Erythrocyte Production}} \text{Red Blood Cells} \tag{3.10}$$

Erythropoiesis is regulated by the interplay of erythropoietin and iron availability, influencing the production of red blood cells.

Thrombopoiesis:

$$\text{Thrombopoietin (TPO)} \xleftrightarrow{\text{Megakaryocyte Maturation}} \text{Platelets} \tag{3.11}$$

Thrombopoiesis involves thrombopoietin driving the maturation of megakaryocytes, leading to the production of platelets.

Mathematical Model:

$$\text{Rate of Hematopoiesis} = k \times \left(\frac{\text{Concentration of Stimulating Factors}}{\text{Inhibiting Factors}} \right) \tag{3.12}$$

A mathematical model relates the rate of hematopoiesis to the balance between stimulating and inhibiting factors.

These equations encapsulate the quantitative and molecular aspects of hematopoiesis, offering insights into blood cell formation.

3.4 Hemoglobinopathies

Hemoglobinopathies, genetic disorders affecting hemoglobin, involve complex molecular and biochemical processes. Let's explore key aspects in a fast and memorable way:

Hemoglobin Structure:

$$\text{Hemoglobin (Hb)} = 4 \text{ Subunits } (2\alpha + 2\beta) + \text{Heme Groups} \tag{3.13}$$

Hemoglobin consists of four subunits $(2\alpha + 2\beta)$ and heme groups, essential for oxygen binding.

Sickle Cell Anemia Mutation:

$$\text{Glutamic Acid} \xleftrightarrow{\text{Point Mutation}} \text{Valine} \xleftrightarrow{\text{HbS Formation}} \text{Sickle Hemoglobin (HbS)} \tag{3.14}$$

Sickle cell anemia arises from a point mutation, transforming glutamic acid to valine, leading to the formation of sickle hemoglobin (HbS).

Thalassemia:

$$\text{Reduced } \alpha \text{ or } \beta \text{ Globin Synthesis} \xleftrightarrow{\text{Imbalanced Globin Chains}} \text{Hemoglobin Variants} \tag{3.15}$$

Thalassemia results from reduced α or β globin synthesis, leading to imbalanced globin chains and the formation of abnormal hemoglobin variants.

Mathematical Analysis:

$$\text{Hemoglobin Variant Percentage} = \frac{\text{Abnormal Hemoglobin}}{\text{Total Hemoglobin}} \times 100\% \tag{3.16}$$

Mathematical analysis involves calculating the percentage of abnormal hemoglobin in the total hemoglobin.

These equations provide insights into the structural and genetic aspects of hemoglobinopathies, aiding in understanding and management.

3.5   Bone Marrow Examination

Bone marrow examination is a vital tool for diagnosing hematological disorders. Let's explore key aspects in a fast and memorable way:

Cellularity Assessment:

$$\text{Cellularity} = \frac{\text{Cellular Elements}}{\text{Total Marrow Volume}} \times 100\% \tag{3.17}$$

Evaluate bone marrow cellularity by determining the percentage of cellular elements in the total marrow volume.

Morphological Analysis:

$$\text{Myeloid: Erythroid Ratio} = \frac{\text{Myeloid Cells}}{\text{Erythroid Cells}} \tag{3.18}$$

Assess bone marrow health by calculating the myeloid to erythroid ratio.

Aspiration Biopsy:

$$\text{Aspiration Rate} = \frac{\text{Number of Aspirated Cells}}{\text{Time of Aspiration}} \tag{3.19}$$

Efficiently measure aspiration biopsy performance with the rate of aspirated cells over the time of aspiration.

Mathematical Model:

$$\text{Hematopoietic Activity} = k \times \left(\frac{\text{Stem Cell Concentration}}{\text{Inhibitory Factors}} \right) \tag{3.20}$$

Use a mathematical model to relate hematopoietic activity to the balance between stem cell concentration and inhibitory factors.

These equations offer practical insights for effective bone marrow examination, aiding accurate diagnoses in hematological conditions.

3.6 Transfusion Medicine

Transfusion medicine plays a crucial role in managing blood-related conditions. Let's explore key aspects in a fast and memorable way:

Blood Compatibility:

$$\text{ABO Compatibility} \xleftrightarrow{\text{Antigen-Antibody Reaction}} \text{Safe Transfusion} \tag{3.21}$$

Ensuring ABO compatibility is vital to prevent antigen-antibody reactions and ensure the safety of blood transfusions.

Crossmatching:

$$\text{Recipient's Serum} + \text{Donor's Red Blood Cells} \xleftrightarrow{\text{No Agglutination}} \text{Compatibility} \tag{3.22}$$

Crossmatching involves testing recipient's serum with donor's red blood cells to ensure compatibility and prevent agglutination.

Transfusion Reaction Rate:

$$\text{Transfusion Reaction Rate} = \frac{\text{Number of Reactions}}{\text{Total Number of Transfusions}} \times 100\% \tag{3.23}$$

The transfusion reaction rate is calculated by determining the percentage of adverse reactions among total transfusions.

Mathematical Model:

$$\text{Transfusion Threshold} = \text{Hemoglobin Level} - \text{Desired Hemoglobin Level} \tag{3.24}$$

A mathematical model calculates the transfusion threshold based on the difference between the current and desired hemoglobin levels.

These equations provide quantitative insights into blood transfusions, ensuring safety and optimizing treatment outcomes.

3.7 Clinical Hematology Cases

Clinical hematology cases provide real-world applications of hematological concepts. Let's explore key aspects in a fast and memorable way:

Iron-Deficiency Anemia:

$$\text{Iron Intake} - \text{Iron Loss} \xleftrightarrow{\text{Hemoglobin Synthesis}} \text{Anemia Severity} \tag{3.25}$$

Iron-deficiency anemia severity depends on the balance between iron intake and loss, crucial for hemoglobin synthesis.

Leukemia Classification:

$$\text{Myeloid Leukemia} \xleftrightarrow{\text{Myeloblast Proliferation}} \text{Bone Marrow Infiltration}$$
$$\xleftrightarrow{\text{Peripheral Blood Blast Count}} \text{Classification} \tag{3.26}$$

Leukemia classification involves myeloid leukemia, myeloblast proliferation, bone marrow infiltration, and peripheral blood blast count.

Platelet Disorders:

$$\text{Thrombocytopenia} \xleftrightarrow{\text{Platelet Destruction}} \text{Bleeding Tendency} \tag{3.27}$$

Platelet disorders, like thrombocytopenia, contribute to bleeding tendencies due to increased platelet destruction.

Mathematical Analysis:

$$\text{Reticulocyte Production Index (RPI)} = \frac{\text{Patient's Reticulocyte Count}}{\text{Normal Reticulocyte Count}} \tag{3.28}$$

Mathematical analysis involves calculating the Reticulocyte Production Index (RPI) based on the patient's and normal reticulocyte counts.

These equations bridge theoretical knowledge with practical applications, enhancing understanding and diagnosis in clinical hematology cases.

Chapter 4

Systemic Pathology

4.1 Cardiovascular System

The cardiovascular system is vital for circulation and oxygen transport. Let's explore key aspects in a fast and memorable way:

Cardiac Output:

$$\text{Cardiac Output} = \text{Heart Rate} \times \text{Stroke Volume} \tag{4.1}$$

Cardiac output, the amount of blood pumped by the heart per minute, is the product of heart rate and stroke volume.

Blood Pressure:

$$\text{Blood Pressure} = \text{Cardiac Output} \times \text{Peripheral Resistance} \tag{4.2}$$

Blood pressure is determined by cardiac output and peripheral resistance, influencing the force of blood against vessel walls.

Atherosclerosis Development:

$$\text{LDL Cholesterol} \xleftrightarrow{\text{Oxidation}} \text{Foam Cells} \xleftrightarrow{\text{Plaque Formation}} \text{Atherosclerosis} \tag{4.3}$$

Atherosclerosis develops as LDL cholesterol undergoes oxidation, leading to the formation of foam cells and arterial plaque.

Mathematical Model:

$$\text{Hemodynamic Shear Stress} = \frac{4 \times \text{Blood Viscosity} \times \text{Vessel Radius}}{\text{Blood Flow Rate}} \tag{4.4}$$

Hemodynamic shear stress, affecting vessel integrity, is calculated based on blood viscosity, vessel radius, and blood flow rate.

These equations provide insights into cardiovascular dynamics, offering a foundation for understanding pathologies and optimizing treatment.

4.2　Respiratory System

The respiratory system plays a crucial role in oxygen exchange. Let's explore key aspects in a fast and memorable way:

Ventilation-Perfusion Ratio:

$$\text{V/Q Ratio} = \frac{\text{Alveolar Ventilation}}{\text{Pulmonary Blood Flow}} \tag{4.5}$$

The ventilation-perfusion ratio (V/Q ratio) assesses the efficiency of gas exchange by comparing alveolar ventilation to pulmonary blood flow.

Lung Compliance:

$$\text{Lung Compliance} = \frac{\text{Change in Lung Volume}}{\text{Change in Transpulmonary Pressure}} \tag{4.6}$$

Lung compliance measures the ease with which the lungs expand and is the ratio of the change in lung volume to the change in transpulmonary pressure.

Oxygen-Hemoglobin Dissociation Curve:

$$\text{Hemoglobin Saturation} \xleftrightarrow{\text{Oxygen Binding/Release}} \text{Partial Pressure of Oxygen (PO2)} \tag{4.7}$$

The oxygen-hemoglobin dissociation curve illustrates the relationship between hemoglobin saturation and the partial pressure of oxygen.

Mathematical Model:

$$\text{Alveolar Gas Equation} : \text{PAO2}$$
$$= (\text{Pb - PH2O}) \times \text{FiO2} - \frac{\text{PaCO2}}{R} \tag{4.8}$$

The alveolar gas equation calculates alveolar oxygen tension (PAO2) based on atmospheric pressure, water vapor pressure, inspired oxygen fraction (FiO2), and arterial carbon dioxide tension (PaCO2).

These equations provide insights into respiratory function, aiding in the understanding of pathologies and optimizing treatment strategies.

4.3 Gastrointestinal System

The gastrointestinal system plays a crucial role in digestion and nutrient absorption. Let's explore key aspects in a fast and memorable way:

Digestive Enzymes:

$$\text{Enzyme Activity} = \text{Enzyme Concentration} \times \text{Substrate Availability} \tag{4.9}$$

Digestive enzyme activity depends on the concentration of enzymes and the availability of substrates for digestion.

Intestinal Absorption:

$$\text{Absorption Rate} = \frac{\text{Surface Area} \times \text{Concentration Gradient}}{\text{Membrane Permeability}} \tag{4.10}$$

The rate of intestinal absorption is influenced by surface area, concentration gradient, and membrane permeability.

Gastrointestinal Motility:

$$\text{Motility Index} = \frac{\text{Contractions per Minute}}{\text{Resistance to Flow}} \tag{4.11}$$

Gastrointestinal motility is quantified by the motility index, representing contractions per minute relative to resistance.

Mathematical Model:

$$\text{Nutrient Bioavailability} = \text{Dietary Intake} \times \left(1 - \frac{\text{Losses during Digestion}}{\text{Total Intake}}\right) \tag{4.12}$$

A mathematical model calculates nutrient bioavailability based on dietary intake and losses during digestion.

These equations provide a framework for understanding gastrointestinal function, aiding in the diagnosis and treatment of digestive disorders.

4.4 Genitourinary System

The genitourinary system plays a critical role in excretion and reproduction. Let's explore key aspects in a fast and memorable way:

Renal Filtration:

$$\text{Glomerular Filtration Rate (GFR)} = \frac{\text{Net Filtration Pressure} \times \text{Filtration Coefficient}}{\text{Plasma Osmotic Pressure}} \tag{4.13}$$

GFR is determined by net filtration pressure, filtration coefficient, and plasma osmotic pressure in renal filtration.

Urine Concentration:

$$\text{Countercurrent Multiplier Effect} = \text{Active Transport} \times \text{Descending Limb Permeability} \quad (4.14)$$

Urine concentration is influenced by the countercurrent multiplier effect involving active transport and descending limb permeability.

Reproductive Hormones:

$$\text{Gonadotropin-Releasing Hormone (GnRH)} \xrightarrow{\text{Pituitary Response}} \text{Follicle-Stimulating Hormone (FSH), Luteinizing Hormone (LH)} \quad (4.15)$$

Reproductive hormones, like GnRH, stimulate the pituitary to release FSH and LH, crucial for reproductive function.

Mathematical Model:

$$\text{Renal Blood Flow} = \frac{\text{Renal Arterial Flow}}{1 - \left(\frac{\text{Renal Vascular Resistance}}{\text{Systemic Vascular Resistance}}\right)} \quad (4.16)$$

A mathematical model calculates renal blood flow based on renal arterial flow, renal vascular resistance, and systemic vascular resistance.

These equations offer insights into renal function and reproductive physiology, contributing to the understanding and management of genitourinary pathologies.

4.5   Endocrine System

The endocrine system regulates various physiological processes through hormonal control. Let's explore key aspects in a fast and memorable way:

Hormone Action:

$$\text{Hormone Effect} = \text{Hormone Concentration} \times \text{Target Cell Sensitivity} \quad (4.17)$$

The effect of a hormone is determined by its concentration and the sensitivity of the target cell to that hormone.

Negative Feedback:

$$\text{Hormone Release} \xrightarrow{\text{Physiological Response}} \text{Inhibition of Further Hormone Release} \quad (4.18)$$

Negative feedback mechanisms ensure that the release of a hormone triggers a physiological response, leading to the inhibition of further hormone release.

Hormone Synthesis:

$$\text{Amino Acid-Derived Hormones} \xleftrightarrow{\text{Enzymatic Modification}} \text{Active Hormones} \tag{4.19}$$

Amino acid-derived hormones undergo enzymatic modification to become active hormones, influencing cellular activities.

Mathematical Model:

$$\text{Half-Life of Hormone} = \frac{0.693}{\text{Hormone Clearance Rate}} \tag{4.20}$$

A mathematical model calculates the half-life of a hormone based on its clearance rate.

These equations provide a framework for understanding endocrine function, emphasizing the dynamic interplay between hormones and target cells.

4.6 Nervous System

The nervous system coordinates complex functions within the body. Let's explore key aspects in a fast and memorable way:

Neuronal Action Potential:

$$\text{Membrane Potential Change} = \text{Stimulus Strength} \times \text{Axon Diameter} \tag{4.21}$$

The change in membrane potential during an action potential is influenced by the stimulus strength and axon diameter.

Synaptic Transmission:

$$\text{Neurotransmitter Release Rate} = \frac{\text{Number of Action Potentials}}{\text{Release Probability}} \tag{4.22}$$

The rate of neurotransmitter release is determined by the number of action potentials and the release probability at the synapse.

Neuroplasticity:

$$\text{Synaptic Strengthening} \xleftrightarrow{\text{Long-Term Potentiation (LTP)}} \text{Enhanced Neuronal Communication} \tag{4.23}$$

Neuroplasticity involves synaptic strengthening through processes like Long-Term Potentiation (LTP), leading to enhanced neuronal communication.

Mathematical Model:

$$\text{Propagation Velocity of Action Potential} = \frac{\text{Axon Diameter}}{\text{Membrane Resistance} \times \text{Axon Capacitance}} \quad (4.24)$$

A mathematical model calculates the propagation velocity of an action potential based on axon diameter, membrane resistance, and axon capacitance.

These equations offer insights into the dynamic functioning of the nervous system, bridging physiological principles with mathematical models.

4.7   Musculoskeletal System

The musculoskeletal system supports movement and provides structural integrity. Let's explore key aspects in a fast and memorable way:

Muscle Contraction:

$$\text{Force of Contraction} = \text{Number of Cross-Bridges} \times \text{Force per Cross-Bridge} \quad (4.25)$$

The force of muscle contraction is influenced by the number of cross-bridges formed and the force exerted by each cross-bridge.

Bone Strength:

$$\text{Bone Mineral Density (BMD)} = \frac{\text{Mineral Content}}{\text{Bone Volume}} \quad (4.26)$$

Bone strength is quantified by bone mineral density (BMD), representing mineral content relative to bone volume.

Joint Flexibility:

$$\text{Joint Range of Motion (ROM)} = \text{Flexibility} \times \text{Joint Structure} \quad (4.27)$$

The range of motion in a joint depends on flexibility and the structural components of the joint.

Mathematical Model:

$$\text{Muscle Work} = \text{Force} \times \text{Distance Moved} \quad (4.28)$$

A mathematical model calculates muscle work based on the force exerted and the distance moved during contraction.

These equations provide insights into the biomechanics of the musculoskeletal system, linking physiological principles with mathematical models.

Chapter 5

Clinical Pathology

5.1 Laboratory Diagnostics

Laboratory diagnostics play a crucial role in disease identification and monitoring. Let's explore key aspects in a fast and memorable way:

Diagnostic Sensitivity and Specificity:

$$\text{Sensitivity} = \frac{\text{True Positives}}{\text{True Positives} + \text{False Negatives}}, \quad \text{Specificity}$$
$$= \frac{\text{True Negatives}}{\text{True Negatives} + \text{False Positives}} \tag{5.1}$$

Sensitivity and specificity quantify the accuracy of a diagnostic test in identifying true positive and true negative results.

Positive Predictive Value (PPV) and Negative Predictive Value (NPV):

$$\text{PPV} = \frac{\text{True Positives}}{\text{True Positives} + \text{False Positives}}, \quad \text{NPV}$$
$$= \frac{\text{True Negatives}}{\text{True Negatives} + \text{False Negatives}} \tag{5.2}$$

PPV and NPV assess the probability of a positive or negative test result being accurate.

Laboratory Test Reliability:

$$\text{Reliability} = \frac{\text{Consistent Results}}{\text{Total Number of Tests}} \times 100\% \tag{5.3}$$

The reliability of a laboratory test is measured by the percentage of consistent results over the total number of tests performed.

Mathematical Model:

$$\text{Diagnostic Odds Ratio (DOR)} = \frac{\text{Sensitivity} \times \text{Specificity}}{1 - \text{Sensitivity}} \times \frac{1 - \text{Specificity}}{\text{Sensitivity}} \quad (5.4)$$

A mathematical model, the Diagnostic Odds Ratio (DOR), evaluates the odds of a positive result in diseased versus non-diseased individuals.

These equations provide a framework for understanding the statistical measures and reliability of laboratory diagnostic tests.

5.2 Clinical Enzymology

Clinical enzymology is crucial for diagnosing various diseases. Let's explore key aspects in a fast and memorable way:

Enzyme Kinetics:

$$\text{Reaction Rate} = \text{Enzyme Concentration} \times \text{Substrate Concentration} \times \text{Catalytic Constant} \quad (5.5)$$

The reaction rate in enzymatic reactions is determined by the concentration of enzymes, substrate, and the catalytic constant.

Enzyme Activity Units:

$$\text{Enzyme Activity} = \frac{\text{Amount of Product Formed}}{\text{Time}} \quad (5.6)$$

Enzyme activity is quantified by the amount of product formed per unit of time.

Enzyme Inhibition:

$$\text{Competitive Inhibition : Inhibitor binds to active site,} \quad \text{Non-competitive Inhibition} \quad (5.7)$$
$$\text{: Inhibitor binds to allosteric site}$$

Competitive and non-competitive inhibition mechanisms affect enzyme activity differently.

Mathematical Model:

$$\text{Michaelis-Menten Equation : Reaction Rate}$$
$$= \frac{\text{Maximal Reaction Rate} \times \text{Substrate Concentration}}{\text{Half-Saturation Constant} + \text{Substrate Concentration}} \quad (5.8)$$

The Michaelis-Menten equation describes the relationship between reaction rate, substrate concentration, maximal reaction rate, and half-saturation constant.

These equations offer insights into the kinetics, measurement, and inhibition of enzymes in clinical settings.

5.3　Immunopathology

Immunopathology explores the role of the immune system in disease. Let's explore key aspects in a fast and memorable way:

Immune Response:

$$\text{Immune Response Strength} = \text{Antigen Presentation} \times \text{T-cell Activation} \times \text{B-cell Activation} \tag{5.9}$$

The strength of the immune response depends on efficient antigen presentation, T-cell activation, and B-cell activation.

Immunoglobulin Classes:

$$\text{IgM, IgG, IgA, IgD, IgE} \xleftrightarrow{\text{Class Switching}} \text{Different Immunoglobulin Classes} \tag{5.10}$$

Class switching diversifies the immunoglobulin classes, each playing distinct roles in immune responses.

Immune Tolerance:

$$\text{Self-Tolerance} \xleftrightarrow{\text{Central Tolerance, Peripheral Tolerance}} \text{Prevention of Autoimmunity} \tag{5.11}$$

Immune tolerance mechanisms, including central and peripheral tolerance, prevent the immune system from attacking the body's own cells.

Mathematical Model:

$$\text{Antibody Affinity} = \frac{\text{Rate of Antibody-Antigen Binding}}{\text{Rate of Antibody Dissociation}} \tag{5.12}$$

A mathematical model calculates antibody affinity based on the rate of antibody-antigen binding and dissociation.

These equations provide a foundation for understanding immune responses, immunoglobulin diversity, immune tolerance, and antibody affinity in immunopathology.

5.4　Molecular Pathology

Molecular pathology delves into the molecular basis of diseases. Let's explore key aspects in a fast and memorable way:

Genetic Mutation Impact:

$$\text{Mutation Severity} = \text{Mutation Type} \times \text{Gene Functionality} \tag{5.13}$$

The severity of a genetic mutation is influenced by the type of mutation and the functionality of the affected gene.

Gene Expression Regulation:

$$\text{Transcription Rate} = \text{Promoter Strength} \times \text{Transcription Factor Binding} \tag{5.14}$$

The rate of gene transcription is determined by the strength of the promoter and the binding of transcription factors.

Epigenetic Modifications:

$$\text{DNA Methylation} + \text{Histone Acetylation} \xleftrightarrow{\text{Gene Expression Regulation}} \text{Altered Chromatin Structure} \tag{5.15}$$

Epigenetic modifications, such as DNA methylation and histone acetylation, influence gene expression by altering chromatin structure.

Mathematical Model:

$$\text{Genetic Variation Index} = \frac{\text{Number of Variants}}{\text{Total Population Genes}} \tag{5.16}$$

A mathematical model calculates the genetic variation index based on the number of genetic variants relative to the total population genes.

These equations provide insights into the impact of genetic mutations, gene expression regulation, epigenetic modifications, and a mathematical model for genetic variation in molecular pathology.

5.5   Microbiology in Pathology

Microbiology plays a vital role in understanding and combating diseases. Let's explore key aspects in a fast and memorable way:

Microbial Growth:

$$\text{Growth Rate} = \text{Doubling Time}^{-1} \tag{5.17}$$

The growth rate of microorganisms is inversely proportional to their doubling time.

Antibiotic Efficacy:

$$\text{Minimum Inhibitory Concentration (MIC)} \xleftrightarrow{\text{Antibiotic Exposure}} \text{Bacterial Growth Inhibition} \tag{5.18}$$

MIC quantifies the minimum concentration of an antibiotic needed to inhibit bacterial growth.

Microbial Load:

$$\text{Total Microbial Load} = \sum \text{Individual Microbial Counts} \tag{5.19}$$

The total microbial load is the sum of individual microbial counts in a given sample.

Mathematical Model:

$$\text{Log Reduction} = \log\left(\frac{\text{Initial Microbial Load}}{\text{Final Microbial Load}}\right) \tag{5.20}$$

A mathematical model, the log reduction, assesses the decrease in microbial load after a treatment or intervention.

These equations provide a foundation for understanding microbial growth, antibiotic efficacy, microbial load, and a mathematical model for evaluating interventions in microbiology.

5.6 Serology and Virology

Serology and virology are crucial in diagnosing and understanding viral infections. Let's explore key aspects in a fast and memorable way:

Antibody Titer:

$$\text{Titer} = \frac{\text{Serum Dilution Factor}}{\text{Highest Dilution Resulting in Reaction}} \tag{5.21}$$

The antibody titer represents the reciprocal of the highest serum dilution resulting in a detectable reaction.

Viral Load:

$$\text{Viral Load} = \text{Number of Viral Copies} \times \text{Sample Volume}^{-1} \tag{5.22}$$

Viral load quantifies the concentration of viral particles in a given sample.

Neutralization Assay:

$$\text{Virus} + \text{Serum} \xleftrightarrow{\text{Neutralization}} \text{Inhibition of Viral Infectivity} \tag{5.23}$$

Neutralization assays assess the ability of serum antibodies to inhibit viral infectivity.

Mathematical Model:

$$\text{Viral Replication Rate} = \frac{\text{Change in Viral Load}}{\text{Time}} \tag{5.24}$$

A mathematical model calculates the rate of viral replication based on the change in viral load over time.

These equations provide insights into antibody titers, viral load quantification, neutralization assays, and a mathematical model for viral replication in serology and virology.

5.7   Pathological Investigations in Clinical Cases

Pathological investigations are essential for diagnosing and understanding diseases. Let's explore key aspects in a fast and memorable way:

Diagnostic Accuracy:

$$\text{Accuracy} = \frac{\text{True Positives} + \text{True Negatives}}{\text{Total Number of Cases}} \tag{5.25}$$

The diagnostic accuracy quantifies the percentage of correctly identified cases.

Positive Likelihood Ratio (LR+):

$$\text{LR+} = \frac{\text{Sensitivity}}{1 - \text{Specificity}} \tag{5.26}$$

LR+ assesses the increase in the odds of a positive test result in diseased individuals.

Negative Likelihood Ratio (LR-):

$$\text{LR-} = \frac{1 - \text{Sensitivity}}{\text{Specificity}} \tag{5.27}$$

LR- evaluates the decrease in the odds of a negative test result in non-diseased individuals.

Mathematical Model:

$$\text{Bayes' Theorem : Posterior Probability}$$
$$= \frac{\text{LR+} \times \text{Prior Probability}}{\text{LR+} \times \text{Prior Probability} + \text{LR-} \times (1 - \text{Prior Probability})} \tag{5.28}$$

Bayes' Theorem calculates the posterior probability of a disease given the test result, considering the LR+ and LR-.

These equations provide insights into diagnostic accuracy, likelihood ratios, and Bayes' Theorem for pathological investigations in clinical cases.

Chapter 6

Pathophysiology

6.1   Mechanisms of Disease

Understanding the mechanisms of disease is crucial for effective intervention. Let's explore key aspects in a fast and memorable way:

Cellular Homeostasis:

$$\text{Cellular Stress} \xleftrightarrow{\text{Adaptation}} \text{Homeostasis Maintenance} \tag{6.1}$$

Cells undergo stress and adapt to maintain homeostasis, ensuring normal cellular functions.

Inflammation Process:

$$\text{Inflammation} = \text{Vasodilation} + \text{Increased Vascular Permeability} + \text{Cellular Infiltration} \tag{6.2}$$

The inflammatory response involves vasodilation, increased vascular permeability, and cellular infiltration to eliminate harmful stimuli.

Oxidative Stress:

$$\text{Reactive Oxygen Species (ROS)} + \text{Antioxidant Defense} \xleftrightarrow{\text{Balance}} \text{Cellular Damage Prevention} \tag{6.3}$$

Maintaining a balance between reactive oxygen species and antioxidant defense prevents oxidative stress-induced cellular damage.

Mathematical Model:

$$\text{Risk Assessment} = \frac{\text{Exposure Level} \times \text{Susceptibility}}{\text{Protective Factors}} \tag{6.4}$$

A mathematical model assesses disease risk considering exposure level, susceptibility, and protective factors.

These equations provide insights into cellular homeostasis, the inflammation process, oxidative stress, and a mathematical model for risk assessment in the mechanisms of disease.

6.2　Pathological Basis of Symptoms

Understanding the pathological basis of symptoms is essential for diagnosis and treatment. Let's explore key aspects in a fast and memorable way:

Pain Perception:

$$\text{Pain Intensity} = \text{Nociceptor Activation} \times \text{Pain Transmission} \tag{6.5}$$

The intensity of pain is influenced by the activation of nociceptors and the transmission of pain signals.

Fever Response:

$$\text{Temperature Increase} = \text{Pyrogen Release} \times \text{Hypothalamus Set Point} \tag{6.6}$$

Fever results from the release of pyrogens altering the hypothalamus set point for body temperature.

Fluid Balance Disturbance:

$$\text{Edema Formation} = \text{Capillary Permeability} \times \text{Oncotic Pressure Imbalance} \tag{6.7}$$

Edema formation is influenced by changes in capillary permeability and imbalances in oncotic pressure.

Mathematical Model:

$$\text{Symptom Severity} = \text{Pathological Changes} \times \text{Individual Sensitivity} \tag{6.8}$$

A mathematical model assesses the severity of symptoms based on pathological changes and individual sensitivity.

These equations provide insights into pain perception, the fever response, fluid balance disturbance, and a mathematical model for symptom severity in the pathological basis of symptoms.

6.3　Genetic and Environmental Factors

Understanding the interplay between genetic and environmental factors is crucial for disease susceptibility. Let's explore key aspects in a fast and memorable way:

Genetic Influence:

$$\text{Genetic Risk} = \text{Genetic Variants} \times \text{Inheritance Pattern} \times \text{Penetrance} \tag{6.9}$$

Genetic risk is influenced by the number of genetic variants, inheritance pattern, and the penetrance of those variants.

Environmental Exposure:

$$\text{Exposure Impact} = \text{Intensity of Exposure} \times \text{Duration} \times \text{Individual Susceptibility} \tag{6.10}$$

The impact of environmental exposure depends on the intensity, duration, and individual susceptibility.

Gene-Environment Interaction:

$$\text{Disease Risk} = \text{Genetic Risk} + \text{Environmental Exposure Impact} + \text{Interaction Terms} \tag{6.11}$$

Disease risk is a result of the combined influence of genetic risk, environmental exposure impact, and interaction terms.

Mathematical Model:

$$\text{Overall Susceptibility} = \frac{\text{Genetic Risk} + \text{Environmental Exposure Impact}}{\text{Protective Factors}} \tag{6.12}$$

A mathematical model calculates overall susceptibility considering genetic risk, environmental exposure impact, and protective factors.

These equations provide insights into genetic influence, environmental exposure, gene-environment interaction, and a mathematical model for overall susceptibility in the context of genetic and environmental factors.

6.4 Multifactorial Diseases

Multifactorial diseases involve a complex interplay of genetic and environmental factors. Let's explore key aspects in a fast and memorable way:

Heritability:

$$\text{Heritability} = \frac{\text{Genetic Variance}}{\text{Total Variance}} \tag{6.13}$$

Heritability quantifies the proportion of phenotypic variance attributable to genetic factors.

Threshold Model:

$$\text{Disease Risk} = \text{Cumulative Genetic Risk} + \text{Cumulative Environmental Risk} - \text{Threshold} \tag{6.14}$$

The threshold model calculates disease risk based on cumulative genetic and environmental risks compared to a threshold.

Interaction Terms:

$$\text{Gene-Gene Interaction} + \text{Gene-Environment Interaction} \xleftrightarrow{\text{Complex Relationships}} \text{Disease Manifestation} \tag{6.15}$$

Interaction terms involving gene-gene and gene-environment interactions contribute to the complex manifestation of multifactorial diseases.

Mathematical Model:

$$\text{Overall Risk} = \frac{\text{Heritability} \times \text{Genetic Risk} + (1 - \text{Heritability}) \times \text{Environmental Risk}}{\text{Protective Factors}} \tag{6.16}$$

A mathematical model integrates heritability, genetic risk, environmental risk, and protective factors to calculate overall risk.

These equations provide insights into heritability, the threshold model, interaction terms, and a mathematical model for overall risk in multifactorial diseases.

6.5 Epidemiology in Pathology

Epidemiology plays a crucial role in understanding disease patterns and risk factors. Let's explore key aspects in a fast and memorable way:

Incidence Rate:

$$\text{Incidence Rate} = \frac{\text{New Cases}}{\text{Population at Risk}} \times \text{Time} \tag{6.17}$$

The incidence rate quantifies the rate of new cases in a population over a specific time period.

Prevalence:

$$\text{Prevalence} = \frac{\text{Total Cases}}{\text{Total Population}} \tag{6.18}$$

Prevalence represents the proportion of the population affected by a disease at a specific point in time.

Attributable Risk:

$$\text{Attributable Risk} = \text{Risk in Exposed Group} - \text{Risk in Unexposed Group} \tag{6.19}$$

Attributable risk assesses the excess risk associated with a particular exposure.

Mathematical Model:

$$\text{Relative Risk} = \frac{\text{Incidence in Exposed Group}}{\text{Incidence in Unexposed Group}} \tag{6.20}$$

A mathematical model, relative risk, compares the incidence in exposed and unexposed groups.

These equations provide insights into incidence rates, prevalence, attributable risk, and a mathematical model for relative risk in epidemiology within pathology.

6.6 Disease Progression

Understanding disease progression is essential for effective management. Let's explore key aspects in a fast and memorable way:

Exponential Growth Model:

$$\text{Disease Burden} = \text{Initial Size} \times e^{\text{Growth Rate} \times \text{Time}} \tag{6.21}$$

The exponential growth model describes the rapid increase in disease burden over time.

Logistic Growth Model:

$$\text{Sigmoid Curve} = \frac{\text{Maximum Capacity}}{1 + e^{-\text{Growth Rate} \times \text{Time}}} \tag{6.22}$$

The logistic growth model represents a sigmoid curve, indicating the saturation of disease progression.

Acceleration and Deceleration:

$$\text{Acceleration} = \frac{\text{Change in Disease Burden}}{\text{Change in Time}}, \quad \text{Deceleration} = -\frac{\text{Change in Disease Burden}}{\text{Change in Time}} \tag{6.23}$$

Acceleration and deceleration measures the rate of change in disease burden over time.

Mathematical Model:

$$\text{Predicted Progression} = \text{Current State} + \text{Acceleration} \times \text{Future Time} \tag{6.24}$$

A mathematical model predicts disease progression based on the current state, acceleration, and future time.

These equations provide insights into exponential and logistic growth models, acceleration, deceleration, and a mathematical model for predicted progression in disease progression.

6.7 Pathophysiology Case Studies

Pathophysiology case studies provide valuable insights into real-world scenarios. Let's explore key aspects in a fast and memorable way:

Case Severity Index:

$$\text{Case Severity Index} = \frac{\text{Clinical Parameters Score}}{\text{Number of Parameters}} \tag{6.25}$$

The case severity index quantifies the severity of a case based on clinical parameters.

Diagnostic Accuracy:

$$\text{Sensitivity} = \frac{\text{True Positives}}{\text{True Positives} + \text{False Negatives}}, \quad \text{Specificity}$$
$$= \frac{\text{True Negatives}}{\text{True Negatives} + \text{False Positives}} \tag{6.26}$$

Sensitivity and specificity assess the accuracy of diagnostic tests in case studies.

Treatment Response Evaluation:

$$\text{Response Rate} = \frac{\text{Number of Responders}}{\text{Total Number of Cases}} \times 100 \tag{6.27}$$

The response rate evaluates the effectiveness of treatments in case studies.

Mathematical Model:

$$\text{Outcome Prediction} = \text{Baseline Characteristics} + \text{Treatment Effects} + \text{Patient Factors} \tag{6.28}$$

A mathematical model predicts outcomes by considering baseline characteristics, treatment effects, and patient factors.

These equations provide insights into case severity index, diagnostic accuracy, treatment response evaluation, and a mathematical model for outcome prediction in pathophysiology case studies.

Chapter 7

Clinical Biochemistry

7.1 Principles of Clinical Biochemistry

Understanding the principles of clinical biochemistry is fundamental for diagnostic processes. Let's explore key aspects in a fast and memorable way:

Enzyme Kinetics:

$$\text{Reaction Velocity} = \text{Maximal Velocity} \times \frac{\text{Substrate Concentration}}{\text{Michaelis-Menten Constant} + \text{Substrate Concentration}} \tag{7.1}$$

Enzyme kinetics describes the rate of biochemical reactions using the Michaelis-Menten equation.

Henderson-Hasselbalch Equation:

$$\text{pH} = \text{pKa} + \log\left(\frac{\text{Conjugate Base}}{\text{Weak Acid}}\right) \tag{7.2}$$

The Henderson-Hasselbalch equation relates the pH of a solution to the pKa and the concentrations of the conjugate base and weak acid.

Beer-Lambert Law:

$$\text{Absorbance} = \varepsilon \times \text{Path Length} \times \text{Concentration} \tag{7.3}$$

The Beer-Lambert Law quantifies the relationship between absorbance, molar absorptivity, path length, and concentration in spectrophotometry.

Mathematical Model:

$$\text{Diagnostic Score} = \sum \left(\text{Weight}_i \times \text{Test Result}_i\right) \tag{7.4}$$

A mathematical model combines weighted test results to generate a diagnostic score.

These equations provide insights into enzyme kinetics, Henderson-Hasselbalch equation, Beer-Lambert Law, and a mathematical model for diagnostic scoring in the principles of clinical biochemistry.

7.2 Biochemical Investigations in Disease

Biochemical investigations are crucial for understanding and diagnosing diseases. Let's explore key aspects in a fast and memorable way:

Diagnostic Sensitivity and Specificity:

$$\text{Sensitivity} = \frac{\text{True Positives}}{\text{True Positives} + \text{False Negatives}}, \quad \text{Specificity} = \frac{\text{True Negatives}}{\text{True Negatives} + \text{False Positives}} \tag{7.5}$$

Sensitivity and specificity measure the accuracy of a diagnostic test in identifying true positives and true negatives.

Positive and Negative Predictive Values:

$$\text{Positive Predictive Value} = \frac{\text{True Positives}}{\text{True Positives} + \text{False Positives}}, \quad \text{Negative Predictive Value} = \frac{\text{True Negatives}}{\text{True Negatives} + \text{False Negatives}} \tag{7.6}$$

Positive and negative predictive values assess the probability of a positive or negative result being correct.

Receiver Operating Characteristic (ROC) Curve:

$$\text{Area under the ROC Curve (AUC)} = \frac{1}{2} \int_0^1 (\text{Sensitivity} + \text{Specificity}) \, d\text{Threshold} \tag{7.7}$$

The ROC curve and AUC provide a visual representation of a diagnostic test's performance.

Mathematical Model:

$$\text{Disease Probability} = \frac{1}{1 + e^{-(\beta_0 + \beta_1 \times \text{Test Result})}} \tag{7.8}$$

A mathematical model predicts the probability of disease based on test results using logistic regression coefficients.

These equations provide insights into diagnostic sensitivity, specificity, predictive values, ROC curve, and a mathematical model for disease probability in biochemical investigations.

7.3 Metabolic Disorders

Metabolic disorders involve disruptions in normal biochemical processes. Let's explore key aspects in a fast and memorable way:

Energy Balance Equation:

$$\text{Energy Intake} = \text{Basal Metabolic Rate (BMR)} + \text{Physical Activity} + \text{Thermic Effect of Food (TEF)} \tag{7.9}$$

The energy balance equation explains the relationship between energy intake, BMR, physical activity, and TEF.

Basal Metabolic Rate (BMR):

Harris-Benedict Equation $\tag{7.10}$

$$: \begin{cases} \text{For Men:} & \text{BMR} = 88.362 + (13.397 \times \text{Weight in kg}) + (4.799 \times \text{Height in cm}) - (5.677 \times \text{Age}) \\ \text{For Women:} & \text{BMR} = 447.593 + (9.247 \times \text{Weight in kg}) + (3.098 \times \text{Height in cm}) - (4.330 \times \text{Age}) \end{cases}$$

The Harris-Benedict equation estimates BMR based on weight, height, and age.

Glycolysis Pathway:

$$\text{Glucose} \xrightarrow{\text{Glycolysis}} \text{Pyruvate} \xrightarrow{\text{Krebs Cycle}} \text{ATP} \tag{7.11}$$

The glycolysis pathway describes the breakdown of glucose to produce ATP in cellular respiration.

Mathematical Model:

$$\text{Metabolic Rate} = \text{BMR} + (\text{Physical Activity Level} \times \text{BMR}) + \text{TEF} \tag{7.12}$$

A mathematical model calculates the total metabolic rate incorporating BMR, physical activity, and TEF.

These equations provide insights into the energy balance equation, Harris-Benedict equation, glycolysis pathway, and a mathematical model for metabolic rate in metabolic disorders.

7.4 Endocrinology in Clinical Biochemistry

Endocrinology plays a crucial role in clinical biochemistry. Let's explore key aspects in a fast and memorable way:

Hormone Regulation:

$$\text{Negative Feedback Loop:} \quad \text{Hormone Release} \xrightarrow{\text{Response}} \text{Inhibition of Further Release} \tag{7.13}$$

Negative feedback loops regulate hormone release to maintain homeostasis.

Hormone Concentration and Receptor Binding:

$$\text{Affinity} = \frac{\text{Hormone-Receptor Binding}}{\text{Hormone Concentration}} \tag{7.14}$$

Affinity measures the strength of hormone-receptor binding relative to hormone concentration.

Insulin and Glucose Homeostasis:

$$\text{Glucose Uptake} \xrightarrow{\text{Insulin}} \text{Glycogenesis} \xrightarrow{\text{Storage}} \text{Maintenance of Blood Glucose Levels} \tag{7.15}$$

Insulin plays a key role in glucose uptake, glycogenesis, and maintaining blood glucose levels.

Thyroid Hormone Regulation:

$$\text{Thyroxine (T4)} \xrightarrow{\text{Conversion}} \text{Triiodothyronine (T3)} \xrightarrow{\text{Negative Feedback}} \text{Hypothalamus and Pituitary} \tag{7.16}$$

Thyroid hormones, T4 and T3, are regulated by a negative feedback loop involving the hypothalamus and pituitary.

Mathematical Model:

$$\text{Hormone Action} = \text{Receptor Binding} \times \left(\frac{\text{Concentration}}{\text{Affinity}} \right) \tag{7.17}$$

A mathematical model describes hormone action by considering receptor binding, concentration, and affinity.

These equations provide insights into negative feedback loops, hormone-receptor binding, insulin and glucose homeostasis, thyroid hormone regulation, and a mathematical model for hormone action in endocrinology.

7.5   Tumor Markers

Tumor markers are vital in diagnosing and monitoring cancer. Let's explore key aspects in a fast and memorable way:

Sensitivity and Specificity of Tumor Markers:

$$\text{Sensitivity} = \frac{\text{True Positives}}{\text{True Positives} + \text{False Negatives}}, \quad \text{Specificity}$$
$$= \frac{\text{True Negatives}}{\text{True Negatives} + \text{False Positives}} \tag{7.18}$$

Sensitivity and specificity assess the accuracy of tumor markers in identifying true positives and true negatives.

Positive Predictive Value (PPV) and Negative Predictive Value (NPV):

$$\text{PPV} = \frac{\text{True Positives}}{\text{True Positives} + \text{False Positives}}, \quad \text{NPV} = \frac{\text{True Negatives}}{\text{True Negatives} + \text{False Negatives}} \tag{7.19}$$

PPV and NPV evaluate the probability of a positive or negative result being correct.

Receiver Operating Characteristic (ROC) Curve:

$$\text{Area under the ROC Curve (AUC)} = \frac{1}{2} \int_0^1 (\text{Sensitivity} + \text{Specificity}) \, d\text{Threshold} \tag{7.20}$$

The ROC curve and AUC visually represent the performance of tumor markers.

Mathematical Model:

$$\text{Risk Prediction} = \frac{1}{1 + e^{-(\beta_0 + \beta_1 \times \text{Tumor Marker Level})}} \tag{7.21}$$

A mathematical model predicts the risk of cancer based on the level of tumor markers using logistic regression coefficients.

These equations provide insights into sensitivity, specificity, PPV, NPV, ROC curve, and a mathematical model for risk prediction in tumor markers.

7.6 Clinical Biochemistry Laboratory Techniques

Clinical biochemistry laboratory techniques are essential for diagnostics. Let's explore key aspects in a fast and memorable way:

Enzyme-Linked Immunosorbent Assay (ELISA):

$$\text{Concentration} = \frac{\text{Absorbance of Sample}}{\text{Absorbance of Standard}} \times \text{Concentration of Standard} \tag{7.22}$$

ELISA calculates the concentration of a substance in a sample based on absorbance measurements and a standard curve.

Polymerase Chain Reaction (PCR):

$$\text{Amplification} = \text{Initial Amount} \times (1 + \text{Amplification Factor})^{\text{Number of Cycles}} \tag{7.23}$$

PCR amplifies DNA exponentially, and the amplification formula shows the increase in the initial amount over cycles.

Chromatography Equation:

$$\text{Retention Time} = \frac{\text{Distance Traveled by Component}}{\text{Distance Traveled by Solvent}} \tag{7.24}$$

Chromatography measures the retention time of components, helping identify substances in a mixture.

Clinical Sensitivity and Specificity:

$$\text{Sensitivity} = \frac{\text{True Positives}}{\text{True Positives} + \text{False Negatives}}, \quad \text{Specificity}$$
$$= \frac{\text{True Negatives}}{\text{True Negatives} + \text{False Positives}} \tag{7.25}$$

Clinical sensitivity and specificity assess the accuracy of laboratory techniques in identifying true positives and true negatives.

Mathematical Model:

$$\text{Laboratory Index} = \sum \left(\text{Weight}_i \times \text{Test Result}_i\right) \tag{7.26}$$

A mathematical model combines weighted test results to generate a laboratory index.

These equations provide insights into ELISA, PCR, chromatography, clinical sensitivity, specificity, and a mathematical model for a laboratory index in clinical biochemistry laboratory techniques.

7.7 Interpretation of Biochemical Data in Clinical Cases

Interpreting biochemical data in clinical cases is essential for diagnosis. Let's explore key aspects in a fast and memorable way:

Renal Function Assessment:

$$\text{Glomerular Filtration Rate (GFR)} = \frac{k \times \text{Creatinine}}{\text{Age}} \tag{7.27}$$

The GFR equation provides an estimate of kidney function, crucial for assessing renal health.

Liver Enzyme Ratios:

$$\text{AST/ALT Ratio} = \frac{\text{AST Level}}{\text{ALT Level}}, \quad \text{Alkaline Phosphatase/ALT Ratio}$$
$$= \frac{\text{ALP Level}}{\text{ALT Level}} \tag{7.28}$$

Ratios of liver enzymes help identify patterns and differentiate between various liver disorders.

Lipid Profile Calculation:

$$\text{Total Cholesterol} = \text{HDL Cholesterol} + \text{LDL Cholesterol} + \frac{\text{Triglycerides}}{5} \tag{7.29}$$

Calculating the total cholesterol level aids in assessing cardiovascular risk.

Diabetes Risk Score:

$$\text{Diabetes Risk Score} = \frac{\text{Fasting Blood Glucose}}{\text{HDL Cholesterol}} \times \frac{\text{Triglycerides}}{2.2} \tag{7.30}$$

The diabetes risk score helps identify individuals at risk for diabetes based on biochemical parameters.

Calcium-Phosphorus Product:

$$\text{Ca} \times \text{P Product} = \text{Serum Calcium} \times \text{Serum Phosphorus} \tag{7.31}$$

Assessing the calcium-phosphorus product is crucial in managing disorders related to mineral metabolism.

These equations provide insights into renal function assessment, liver enzyme ratios, lipid profile calculation, diabetes risk score, and calcium-phosphorus product in interpreting biochemical data in clinical cases.

Chapter 8

Pathology of Infectious Diseases

8.1 Bacterial Infections

Understanding bacterial infections is crucial. Let's explore key aspects in a fast and memorable way:

Bacterial Growth Rate:

$$\text{Growth Rate} = \frac{\text{Final Bacterial Population} - \text{Initial Bacterial Population}}{\text{Initial Bacterial Population} \times \text{Time}} \tag{8.1}$$

The growth rate equation quantifies how rapidly bacteria multiply over time.

Minimum Inhibitory Concentration (MIC):

$$\text{MIC} = \text{Lowest Concentration of Antibiotic Inhibiting Bacterial Growth} \tag{8.2}$$

MIC is a crucial parameter in determining the effectiveness of antibiotics against bacterial infections.

Bacterial Virulence Factors:

$$\text{Virulence Index} = \frac{\text{Expression of Virulence Factors}}{\text{Bacterial Load}} \tag{8.3}$$

The virulence index assesses the relationship between virulence factor expression and bacterial load.

Bacterial Reproduction Model:

$$\frac{dN}{dt} = rN\left(1 - \frac{N}{K}\right) - dN \tag{8.4}$$

A logistic growth model describes the dynamics of bacterial population, considering factors like carrying capacity (K) and death rate (d).

Bacterial Biofilm Formation:

$$\text{Biofilm Formation Rate} = \frac{\text{Biofilm Biomass}}{\text{Time}} \tag{8.5}$$

Understanding biofilm formation is crucial in managing chronic bacterial infections.

These equations provide insights into bacterial growth rate, minimum inhibitory concentration (MIC), bacterial virulence factors, a bacterial reproduction model, and biofilm formation in bacterial infections.

8.2   Viral Infections

Understanding viral infections is crucial. Let's explore key aspects in a fast and memorable way:

Viral Replication Cycle:

$$\text{Virus Replication Rate} = \frac{\text{Final Viral Load} - \text{Initial Viral Load}}{\text{Initial Viral Load} \times \text{Time}} \tag{8.6}$$

The virus replication rate quantifies how rapidly viruses multiply within a host.

Viral Load Dynamics:

$$\frac{dV}{dt} = rV\left(1 - \frac{V}{K}\right) - cV \tag{8.7}$$

A logistic growth model describes the dynamics of viral load, considering factors like carrying capacity (K) and clearance rate (c).

Antiviral Drug Half-life:

$$\text{Drug Half-life} = \frac{0.693}{\text{Elimination Rate Constant}} \tag{8.8}$$

Understanding the half-life of antiviral drugs is crucial for dosing regimens and treatment efficacy.

Viral Mutation Rate:

$$\text{Mutation Rate} = \frac{\text{Number of Mutations}}{\text{Total Viral Replication}} \tag{8.9}$$

The viral mutation rate influences the adaptability and evolution of viruses.

Virus-Host Interaction Index:

$$\text{Interaction Index} = \frac{\text{Viral Receptor Binding Affinity}}{\text{Host Immune Response Strength}} \tag{8.10}$$

Assessing the interaction index provides insights into the balance between virus and host factors.

These equations provide insights into viral replication rate, viral load dynamics, antiviral drug half-life, viral mutation rate, and virus-host interaction index in viral infections.

8.3 Parasitic Infections

Understanding parasitic infections is crucial. Let's explore key aspects in a fast and memorable way:

Parasite Life Cycle:

$$\text{Life Cycle Duration} = \frac{\text{Time for Complete Life Cycle}}{\text{Number of Reproductive Cycles}} \tag{8.11}$$

The duration of the parasite life cycle provides insights into its reproduction patterns.

Parasite Load Dynamics:

$$\frac{dP}{dt} = rP\left(1 - \frac{P}{K}\right) - cP \tag{8.12}$$

A logistic growth model describes the dynamics of parasite load, considering factors like carrying capacity (K) and clearance rate (c).

Parasitic Resistance Mutation Rate:

$$\text{Mutation Rate} = \frac{\text{Number of Resistance Mutations}}{\text{Total Parasitic Replication}} \tag{8.13}$$

Understanding the mutation rate is crucial in assessing the development of resistance to antiparasitic drugs.

Antiparasitic Drug Half-life:

$$\text{Drug Half-life} = \frac{0.693}{\text{Elimination Rate Constant}} \tag{8.14}$$

Understanding the half-life of antiparasitic drugs is crucial for dosing regimens and treatment efficacy.

Parasite-Host Interaction Index:

$$\text{Interaction Index} = \frac{\text{Parasite Attachment Strength}}{\text{Host Immune Response Intensity}} \tag{8.15}$$

Assessing the interaction index provides insights into the balance between parasite and host factors.

These equations provide insights into parasite life cycle duration, parasite load dynamics, parasitic resistance mutation rate, antiparasitic drug half-life, and parasite-host interaction index in parasitic infections.

8.4 Fungal Infections

Understanding fungal infections is crucial. Let's explore key aspects in a fast and memorable way:

Fungal Growth Rate:

$$\text{Growth Rate} = \frac{\text{Final Fungal Population} - \text{Initial Fungal Population}}{\text{Initial Fungal Population} \times \text{Time}} \tag{8.16}$$

The growth rate equation quantifies how rapidly fungi multiply over time.

Fungal Load Dynamics:

$$\frac{dF}{dt} = rF\left(1 - \frac{F}{K}\right) - cF \tag{8.17}$$

A logistic growth model describes the dynamics of fungal load, considering factors like carrying capacity (K) and clearance rate (c).

Fungal Resistance Mutation Rate:

$$\text{Mutation Rate} = \frac{\text{Number of Resistance Mutations}}{\text{Total Fungal Replication}} \tag{8.18}$$

Understanding the mutation rate is crucial in assessing the development of resistance to antifungal drugs.

Antifungal Drug Half-life:

$$\text{Drug Half-life} = \frac{0.693}{\text{Elimination Rate Constant}} \tag{8.19}$$

Understanding the half-life of antifungal drugs is crucial for dosing regimens and treatment efficacy.

Fungus-Host Interaction Index:

$$\text{Interaction Index} = \frac{\text{Fungal Adhesion Strength}}{\text{Host Immune Response Potency}} \tag{8.20}$$

Assessing the interaction index provides insights into the balance between fungus and host factors.

These equations provide insights into fungal growth rate, fungal load dynamics, fungal resistance mutation rate, antifungal drug half-life, and fungus-host interaction index in fungal infections.

8.5 Emerging Infectious Diseases

Understanding emerging infectious diseases is crucial. Let's explore key aspects in a fast and memorable way:

Basic Reproduction Number (R_0):

$$R_0 = \text{Transmission Rate} \times \text{Duration of Infectiousness} \tag{8.21}$$

The basic reproduction number quantifies the potential for disease spread within a population.

Epidemic Growth Rate:

$$\text{Growth Rate} = \frac{\text{Final Epidemic Size} - \text{Initial Epidemic Size}}{\text{Initial Epidemic Size} \times \text{Time}} \tag{8.22}$$

The growth rate equation describes the rate of increase in the size of an epidemic.

Effective Reproduction Number (R_t):

$$R_t = R_0 \times \left(1 - \frac{\text{Proportion of Immune Population}}{\text{Total Population}}\right) \tag{8.23}$$

The effective reproduction number considers the proportion of the population with immunity.

Outbreak Probability:

$$\text{Probability} = 1 - \exp\left(-R_t \times \text{Time}\right) \tag{8.24}$$

The outbreak probability estimates the likelihood of an epidemic.

Disease Spread Rate:

$$\frac{dI}{dt} = \beta I \left(1 - \frac{I}{K}\right) - \gamma I \tag{8.25}$$

A logistic growth model describes the dynamics of disease spread, considering factors like carrying capacity (K) and recovery rate (γ).

These equations provide insights into R_0, epidemic growth rate, R_t, outbreak probability, and disease spread rate in emerging infectious diseases.

8.6 Infection Control Measures

Effectively controlling infectious diseases is crucial. Let's explore key aspects in a fast and memorable way:

Basic Reproduction Number (R_0):

$$R_0 = \frac{\text{Transmission Rate}}{\text{Recovery Rate}} \tag{8.26}$$

The basic reproduction number helps assess the potential for disease spread in a population.

Herd Immunity Threshold:

$$\text{Herd Immunity} = 1 - \frac{1}{R_0} \tag{8.27}$$

Understanding the herd immunity threshold is crucial for vaccination strategies and disease control.

Transmission Dynamics:

$$\frac{dI}{dt} = \beta I \left(1 - \frac{I}{N}\right) - \gamma I \tag{8.28}$$

A compartmental model describes the transmission dynamics, considering factors like contact rate (β) and recovery rate (γ).

Effective Reproduction Number (R_{eff}):

$$R_{\text{eff}} = R_0 \left(1 - \frac{1}{\text{Intervention Effectiveness}}\right) \tag{8.29}$$

The effective reproduction number accounts for the impact of intervention measures.

Isolation Compliance Rate:

$$\text{Compliance Rate} = \frac{\text{Number of Compliant Individuals}}{\text{Total Isolated Individuals}} \tag{8.30}$$

Assessing isolation compliance is crucial for the success of quarantine measures.

These equations provide insights into infection control measures, including R_0, herd immunity threshold, transmission dynamics, R_{eff}, and isolation compliance rate.

8.7 Clinical Cases in Infectious Disease Pathology

In this section, we explore key aspects of clinical cases in infectious disease pathology, presenting information in a fast and memorable way.

Epidemiological Measures:

$$\text{Attack Rate} = \frac{\text{Number of new cases}}{\text{Population at risk}} \times 100$$

$$\text{Incidence Rate} = \frac{\text{Number of new cases}}{\text{Population at risk}} \times 1000$$

Disease Transmission Model:

$$\frac{dI}{dt} = \beta I \left(1 - \frac{I}{N}\right) - \gamma I$$

This model describes the transmission dynamics of infectious diseases in a population, considering the susceptible (S), infected (I), and recovered (R) compartments.

Basic Reproduction Number (R_0):

$$R_0 = \frac{\beta}{\gamma}$$

R_0 represents the average number of secondary infections produced by one infected individual in a completely susceptible population.

SIR Model Equations:

$$\frac{dS}{dt} = -\beta \frac{SI}{N}$$

$$\frac{dI}{dt} = \beta \frac{SI}{N} - \gamma I$$

$$\frac{dR}{dt} = \gamma I$$

These equations represent the Susceptible-Infectious-Recovered (SIR) model.

Contact Number (C):

$$C = \frac{\text{Number of contacts per unit time}}{\text{Probability of disease transmission per contact}}$$

Understanding the contact number is crucial for assessing the potential for disease spread.

Mathematical Formulas in Molecular Biology:

$$DNA \rightarrow RNA$$
$$\rightarrow \text{Protein}$$

This represents the central dogma of molecular biology.

Utilizing these mathematical models and equations enhances our understanding of the epidemiology and dynamics of infectious diseases, aiding in the analysis of clinical cases.

Chapter 9

Environmental and Nutritional Pathology

9.1 Environmental Factors in Disease

In this section, we explore the impact of environmental factors on disease, presenting information in a fast and memorable way.

Environmental Risk Assessment:

$$\text{Risk} = \text{Hazard} \times \text{Exposure}$$

Understanding the risk associated with environmental hazards is crucial for disease prevention.

Air Quality Index (AQI):

$$AQI = \frac{1}{N} \sum_{i=1}^{N} \left(\frac{C_i}{I_i} \right)$$

The AQI provides a numerical scale for reporting air quality and associated health effects.

Water Quality Index (WQI):

$$WQI = \left(\sum_{i=1}^{n} w_i \times \frac{p_i}{s_i} \right) \times 100$$

WQI is a measure of water quality that considers various parameters.

Chemical Exposure Pathways:

$$\text{Exposure} = \text{Concentration} \times \text{Time}$$

Chemical exposure pathways play a role in the development of environmentally related diseases.

Foodborne Pathogen Risk Assessment:

$$\text{Risk} = \text{Hazard} \times \text{Exposure} \times \text{Consequence}$$

Assessing the risk of foodborne pathogens involves considering the hazard, exposure, and potential consequences.

Chemical Equation for Environmental Transformation:

$$A \xrightarrow{\text{Environmental Factors}} B$$

Environmental factors can lead to transformations in chemical substances, influencing disease patterns.

Nutritional Impact on Disease:

$$\text{Nutrient Intake} = \frac{\text{Amount Consumed}}{\text{Body Weight}}$$

Balanced nutrition is essential for maintaining health and preventing nutritional diseases.

Molecular Equation for Nutrient Absorption:

$$Nutrient_{\text{in food}} + Enzymes \rightarrow AbsorbedNutrient$$

Understanding the molecular processes of nutrient absorption is key to addressing nutritional pathology.

These mathematical formulations provide insights into the assessment and impact of environmental and nutritional factors on disease, aiding in the development of preventive strategies.

9.2   Nutritional Deficiencies

In this section, we explore nutritional deficiencies, presenting information in a fast and memorable way.

Essential Nutrients:

$$\text{Essential Nutrient} = \text{Nutrient that must be obtained from diet}$$

Understanding essential nutrients is crucial for preventing nutritional deficiencies.

Recommended Dietary Allowance (RDA):

$$RDA = \text{Average daily nutrient intake sufficient to meet the requirements of nearly all individuals}$$

The RDA provides guidelines for optimal nutrient intake to prevent deficiencies.

Malnutrition Index:

$$\text{Malnutrition Index} = \frac{\text{Actual Intake}}{\text{Required Intake}} \times 100$$

Assessing the malnutrition index helps identify individuals at risk of nutritional deficiencies.

Biochemical Markers of Nutritional Status:

$$\text{Nutrient Blood Level} \xrightarrow{\text{Deficiency}} \text{Abnormal Biochemical Marker}$$

Biochemical markers play a role in diagnosing nutritional deficiencies.

Iron Deficiency Anemia Equation:

$$\text{Hemoglobin} \xrightarrow{\text{Iron Deficiency}} \text{Reduced Hemoglobin Levels}$$

Iron deficiency is a common cause of anemia, impacting hemoglobin levels.

Vitamin Deficiency Molecular Equation:

$$\text{Vitamin} + \text{Enzyme} \xrightarrow{\text{Deficiency}} \text{Inhibited Enzymatic Reactions}$$

Vitamin deficiencies can lead to inhibited enzymatic reactions, affecting various physiological processes.

Calcium Deficiency Equation:

$$\text{Calcium Intake} \xrightarrow{\text{Deficiency}} \text{Reduced Bone Mineral Density}$$

Calcium deficiency is associated with decreased bone mineral density and increased risk of fractures.

Zinc Deficiency Equation:

$$\text{Zinc} \xrightarrow{\text{Deficiency}} \text{Impaired Immune Function}$$

Zinc deficiency can impair immune function, leading to increased susceptibility to infections.

These mathematical formulations provide insights into the assessment and impact of nutritional deficiencies, aiding in the development of strategies for optimal nutrition.

9.3   Toxicology and Pathology

In this section, we delve into Toxicology and its intersection with Pathology, presenting information in a fast and memorable way.

Toxicology Overview:

$$\text{Toxicology} = \text{Study of harmful effects of substances on living organisms}$$

Understanding toxicology is essential for assessing the impact of various substances on health.

Dose-Response Relationship:

$$\text{Response} \xrightarrow{\text{Increases with}} \text{Dose of Toxic Substance}$$

Establishing the dose-response relationship helps determine the toxicity level of a substance.

LD50 (Lethal Dose 50):

$$\text{LD50} = \text{Dose at which 50\% of exposed individuals die}$$

LD50 is a crucial measure in toxicology to assess the lethal dose of a substance.

Toxicokinetics Equation:

$$\text{Toxicokinetics} = \frac{\text{Absorption} \times \text{Distribution}}{\text{Metabolism} + \text{Excretion}}$$

Understanding toxicokinetics helps predict the fate of toxic substances within the body.

Metabolic Activation Equation:

$$\text{Pro-toxin} \xrightarrow{\text{Metabolic Activation}} \text{Toxic Metabolite}$$

Metabolic activation can transform pro-toxins into toxic metabolites, influencing toxicity.

Organ Toxicity Equation:

$$\text{Toxic Substance} \xrightarrow{\text{Accumulation}} \text{Organ-Specific Toxicity}$$

Certain substances may accumulate in specific organs, leading to organ-specific toxicity.

Carcinogenesis Pathway:

$$\text{Initiation} \xrightarrow{\text{Promotion}} \text{Progression} \xrightarrow{\text{Cancer}}$$

Understanding the carcinogenesis pathway is crucial for assessing the potential of substances to induce cancer.

Chemical Exposure Risks:

$$\text{Risk} = \text{Exposure} \times \text{Toxicity}$$

Evaluating chemical exposure risks involves considering both exposure levels and the toxicity of substances.

These mathematical formulations provide insights into the complex relationship between toxicology and pathology, aiding in the assessment of the impact of toxic substances on living organisms.

9.4 Malnutrition and Disease

In this section, we delve into the relationship between malnutrition and disease, presenting information in a fast and memorable way.

Malnutrition Impact Equation:

$$\text{Malnutrition Impact} = \text{Poor Nutrition} \times \text{Increased Disease Susceptibility}$$

Understanding the impact of malnutrition involves considering its role in increasing susceptibility to various diseases.

Protein-Energy Malnutrition (PEM) Equation:

$$\text{PEM} = \text{Inadequate Protein Intake} + \text{Inadequate Caloric Intake}$$

PEM results from insufficient protein and caloric intake, contributing to a range of health issues.

Effects of Micronutrient Deficiencies:

$$\text{Micronutrient Deficiency} \xrightarrow{\text{Impact on Immune System}} \text{Reduced Immune Function}$$

Micronutrient deficiencies, such as vitamin and mineral deficiencies, can compromise immune function.

Malnutrition and Gastrointestinal Diseases Equation:

$$\text{Malnutrition} \xrightarrow{\text{Gastrointestinal Diseases}} \text{Impaired Nutrient Absorption}$$

Gastrointestinal diseases associated with malnutrition can lead to impaired nutrient absorption, exacerbating nutritional deficiencies.

Metabolic Consequences of Malnutrition:

$$\text{Malnutrition} \xrightarrow{\text{Metabolic Disturbances}} \text{Energy Imbalance}$$

Malnutrition contributes to metabolic disturbances, resulting in an energy imbalance with profound health consequences.

Malnutrition and Cardiovascular Diseases Equation:

$$\text{Malnutrition} \xrightarrow{\text{Cardiovascular Diseases}} \text{Altered Lipid Profile}$$

Malnutrition can impact lipid profiles, contributing to the development of cardiovascular diseases.

Impact of Malnutrition on Neurological Function:

$$\text{Malnutrition} \xrightarrow{\text{Neurological Dysfunction}} \text{Impaired Cognitive Function}$$

Neurological dysfunction resulting from malnutrition can lead to impaired cognitive function.

This section highlights the intricate connections between malnutrition and various diseases, emphasizing the importance of addressing nutritional aspects in disease prevention and management.

9.5   Foodborne Illnesses

In this section, we explore the world of foodborne illnesses, presenting information in a fast and memorable way.

Food Contamination Equation:

$$\text{Food Contamination} = \text{Pathogenic Microorganisms} + \text{Toxins} + \text{Chemical Contaminants}$$

Foodborne illnesses can result from the presence of pathogenic microorganisms, toxins, and chemical contaminants in food.

Microbial Pathogens in Food Equation:

$$\text{Microbial Pathogens} = \text{Bacteria} + \text{Viruses} + \text{Parasites}$$

Various microorganisms, including bacteria, viruses, and parasites, can be responsible for foodborne infections.

Toxin-Producing Microorganisms Equation:

$$\text{Toxin-Producing Microorganisms} \xrightarrow{\text{Toxin Production}} \text{Toxicity}$$

Certain microorganisms have the ability to produce toxins, leading to the toxicity of contaminated food.

Chemical Contaminants in Food Equation:

$$\text{Chemical Contaminants} = \text{Pesticides} + \text{Food Additives} + \text{Heavy Metals}$$

Chemical contaminants, such as pesticides, food additives, and heavy metals, can pose health risks when present in food.

Impact of Foodborne Illnesses on Gastrointestinal Tract:

$$\text{Foodborne Illness} \xrightarrow{\text{Gastrointestinal Symptoms}} \text{Nausea, Vomiting, Diarrhea}$$

Foodborne illnesses often manifest with gastrointestinal symptoms, including nausea, vomiting, and diarrhea.

Immune Response to Foodborne Pathogens:

$$\text{Immune Response} = \text{Antibodies} + \text{Cellular Defense}$$

The body's immune response involves the production of antibodies and cellular defense mechanisms against foodborne pathogens.

Prevention of Foodborne Illnesses Equation:

$$\text{Prevention} = \text{Food Safety Practices} + \text{Proper Food Handling} + \text{Hygiene}$$

Effective prevention of foodborne illnesses requires adherence to food safety practices, proper food handling, and maintaining good hygiene.

This section sheds light on the diverse factors contributing to foodborne illnesses and emphasizes the importance of preventive measures for ensuring food safety.

9.6 Environmental and Nutritional Pathology Investigations

In this section, we delve into the realm of environmental and nutritional pathology investigations, presenting information in a concise and memorable way.

Environmental Pathology Investigation Equation:

$$\text{Environmental Pathology Investigation} = \text{Exposure Assessment} + \text{Toxicity Analysis} + \text{Risk Assessment}$$

Environmental pathology investigations involve assessing exposure to environmental factors, analyzing toxicity, and conducting risk assessments.

Nutritional Pathology Investigation Equation:

$$\text{Nutritional Pathology Investigation} = \text{Dietary Assessment} + \text{Nutrient Analysis} + \text{Metabolic Profiling}$$

Nutritional pathology investigations encompass dietary assessment, nutrient analysis, and metabolic profiling to understand the impact of nutrition on health.

Exposure Assessment in Environmental Pathology:

$$\text{Exposure Assessment} = \text{Environmental Contaminants} + \text{Occupational Exposures} + \text{Residential Exposures}$$

Assessing exposure involves evaluating environmental contaminants, occupational exposures, and exposures related to residence.

Toxicity Analysis Equation:

$$\text{Toxicity Analysis} = \text{Cellular Toxicity} + \text{Organ Toxicity} + \text{Systemic Toxicity}$$

Toxicity analysis explores the impact of environmental factors on cellular, organ, and systemic levels of the body.

Risk Assessment in Environmental Pathology:

$$\text{Risk Assessment} = \text{Hazard Identification} + \text{Dose-Response Assessment} + \text{Exposure Assessment}$$

Risk assessment involves identifying hazards, assessing dose-response relationships, and evaluating exposure to determine potential risks.

Dietary Assessment in Nutritional Pathology:

$$\text{Dietary Assessment} = \text{Food Frequency Questionnaire} + \text{Dietary Recall} + \text{Nutrient Intake Analysis}$$

Evaluating nutrition includes methods such as food frequency questionnaires, dietary recalls, and analysis of nutrient intake.

Nutrient Analysis Equation:

$$\text{Nutrient Analysis} = \text{Macronutrients} + \text{Micronutrients} + \text{Biochemical Markers}$$

Nutrient analysis covers the assessment of macronutrients, micronutrients, and biochemical markers for a comprehensive understanding of nutritional status.

Metabolic Profiling in Nutritional Pathology:

$$\text{Metabolic Profiling} = \text{Metabolites} + \text{Metabolic Pathways} + \text{Biomarkers}$$

Exploring metabolic profiles involves analyzing metabolites, metabolic pathways, and biomarkers associated with nutritional pathways.

This section provides insights into the methodologies used in environmental and nutritional pathology investigations, employing a combination of exposure assessments, toxicity analyses, and risk assessments in environmental pathology, and dietary assessments, nutrient analyses, and metabolic profiling in nutritional pathology.

9.7 Case Studies in Environmental Pathology

In this section, we explore case studies in environmental pathology, presenting information in a concise and memorable way.

Case Study 1: Industrial Pollution Impact

$$\text{Health Impact} = \text{Exposure Level} \times \text{Toxicity} \nabla \cdot \text{Protective Factors}$$

Analyzing the impact of industrial pollution involves assessing exposure levels, toxicity, and protective factors to understand the associated health risks.

Case Study 2: Occupational Hazard Assessment

$$\text{Risk} = \text{Hazard Probability} \times \text{Exposure Duration} \times \text{Individual Susceptibility}$$

Assessing occupational hazards requires evaluating the probability of hazards, exposure duration, and individual susceptibility to determine overall risk.

Case Study 3: Residential Exposure Investigation

$$\text{Exposure Index} = \text{Contaminant Level} \times \text{Exposure Duration} \nabla \cdot \text{Protective Measures}$$

Investigating residential exposures involves calculating exposure indices based on contaminant levels, exposure duration, and the effectiveness of protective measures.

Case Study 4: Ecological Impact Assessment

$$\text{Ecological Impact} = \text{Biodiversity Loss} + \text{Ecosystem Disturbance} + \text{Restoration Potential}$$

Assessing ecological impact considers factors such as biodiversity loss, ecosystem disturbance, and the potential for restoration.

Case Study 5: Environmental Cleanup Cost Estimation

$$\text{Cleanup Cost} = \text{Pollutant Quantity} \times \text{Remediation Cost per Unit} + \text{Site-Specific Factors}$$

Estimating environmental cleanup costs involves calculating the quantity of pollutants, the cost per unit of remediation, and site-specific factors.

Case Study 6: Community Health Risk Perception

$$\text{Risk Perception} = \text{Media Coverage} \times \text{Community Awareness} \times \text{Perceived Severity}$$

Assessing community health risk perception considers factors like media coverage, community awareness, and the perceived severity of the risk.

These case studies provide practical insights into the application of environmental pathology concepts. Each case study utilizes mathematical formulas and equations to quantify various aspects, making the information accessible and memorable.

Chapter 10

Forensic Pathology

10.1 Principles of Forensic Pathology

In this section, we delve into the principles of forensic pathology, presenting information in a concise and memorable way.

Forensic Investigation Timeline:

$$\text{Death Interval} = \text{Postmortem Interval} + \text{Antemortem Interval}$$

Understanding the time of death involves analyzing both the postmortem and antemortem intervals to establish a comprehensive death interval.

Estimation of Stature from Bones:

$$\text{Estimated Stature} = a + b \times \text{Bone Length}$$

Forensic anthropologists use regression equations (a and b are constants) to estimate stature from the length of bones found in forensic cases.

Gunshot Residue Analysis:

$$\text{GSR Ratio} = \frac{\text{Metal Elements}}{\text{Non-Metal Elements}}$$

Analyzing the ratio of metal to non-metal elements in gunshot residue helps determine the proximity of a firearm to a person at the time of discharge.

Bloodstain Pattern Analysis:

$$\text{Angle of Impact} = \arcsin\left(\frac{\text{Width of Bloodstain}}{\text{Length of Bloodstain}}\right)$$

Bloodstain pattern analysts use trigonometry to calculate the angle of impact, providing insights into the dynamics of a crime scene.

DNA Profiling Probability:

$$\text{Probability of Match} = \left(\frac{1}{2}\right)^n$$

Forensic DNA analysts assess the probability of a match between crime scene DNA and a suspect, with n representing the number of loci tested.

Toxicology Analysis:

$$\text{Blood Alcohol Concentration (BAC)} = \frac{\text{Alcohol in Blood}}{\text{Blood Volume}} \times 100$$

Determining blood alcohol concentration involves calculating the ratio of alcohol in the blood to the total blood volume.

These principles and formulas illustrate the quantitative aspects of forensic pathology, aiding forensic investigators in unraveling mysteries surrounding crime scenes.

10.2 Postmortem Examination

In this section, we delve into the intricacies of postmortem examination in forensic pathology, elucidating key concepts through concise and memorable mathematical formulas and equations.

Time Since Death (TSD) Estimation:

$$\text{TSD} = \text{Postmortem Interval} + \text{Antemortem Interval}$$

Forensic investigators determine the time since death by summing the postmortem interval with the antemortem interval.

Rigor Mortis Development:

$$\text{Rigor Mortis Index} = \frac{\text{Number of Joints Stiff}}{\text{Total Number of Joints}} \times 100$$

The rigor mortis index, representing the percentage of stiff joints, offers insights into the progression of rigor mortis.

Decomposition Rate:

$$\text{Decomposition Rate} = \frac{\text{Number of Insects}}{\text{Postmortem Interval}}$$

Forensic pathologists analyze the decomposition rate, calculated as the number of insects per unit postmortem interval, aiding in understanding decay timelines.

Lividity Analysis:

$$\text{Lividity Score} = \frac{\text{Area of Fixed Lividity}}{\text{Total Body Surface Area}} \times 10$$

Lividity scores, derived from the area of fixed lividity relative to the total body surface area, help determine the body's postmortem positioning.

Hydrostatic Testing:

$$\text{Lung Buoyancy} = \frac{\text{Lung Weight in Air}}{\text{Lung Weight in Water}}$$

Hydrostatic testing assesses lung buoyancy, providing clues about drowning incidents and the body's submersion position.

Estimation of Blood Loss:

$$\text{Estimated Blood Loss} = \frac{\text{Volume of Blood in Stomach}}{\text{Hematocrit Value}} \times 100$$

Estimating blood loss involves measuring the volume of blood in the stomach and considering the hematocrit value.

By incorporating these formulas, forensic pathologists enhance their ability to interpret postmortem findings, contributing valuable insights to criminal investigations.

10.3 Identification of Remains

In this section, we explore the methods and mathematical formulations used in the identification of remains in forensic pathology.

Dental Identification:

$$\text{Dental Index} = \frac{\text{Maxillary Tooth Width}}{\text{Mandibular Tooth Width}}$$

Forensic odontologists employ the dental index, comparing the width of maxillary and mandibular teeth, aiding in individual identification.

Cranial Morphology:

$$\text{Cranial Index} = \frac{\text{Maximum Cranial Width}}{\text{Maximum Cranial Length}} \times 100$$

The cranial index, calculated from the ratio of maximum cranial width to length, contributes to skull-based identification.

DNA Profiling:

$$\text{Matching Probability} = 1 - (1 - \text{Matching Rate})^{\text{Number of Loci}}$$

DNA profiling utilizes the matching probability formula to estimate the likelihood of a match across multiple genetic loci.

Facial Reconstruction:

$$\text{Facial Soft Tissue Depth} = \frac{\text{Skull Length} + \text{Skull Width}}{2} \times \text{Specific Facial Depth Coefficient}$$

Facial reconstruction involves estimating facial soft tissue depth based on skull dimensions and specific coefficients.

Postmortem Imaging:

$$\text{Facial Recognition Score} = \frac{\text{Number of Matched Facial Features}}{\text{Total Number of Features}} \times 100$$

Postmortem imaging employs facial recognition scores, reflecting the percentage of matched facial features for identification.

Isotopic Analysis:

$$\text{Isotope Ratio} = \frac{\text{Heavy Isotope Count}}{\text{Total Isotope Count}}$$

Isotopic analysis assists in geographical identification, examining the ratio of heavy isotopes in remains.

By incorporating these formulas, forensic pathologists enhance their ability to identify remains, contributing valuable insights to medico-legal investigations.

10.4   Trauma and Injury Analysis

This section provides a rapid overview of trauma and injury analysis in forensic pathology, emphasizing mathematical formulas and equations for quick comprehension.

Blunt Force Trauma:

$$\text{Impact Force} = \frac{\text{Mass} \times \text{Change in Velocity}}{\text{Time of Impact}}$$

For blunt force trauma, understanding the impact force is crucial, calculated by considering mass, change in velocity, and the duration of impact.

Sharp Force Injuries:

$$\text{Wound Channel Diameter} = \frac{\text{Blade Width} + \text{Soft Tissue Thickness}}{2}$$

Sharp force injuries, such as stabbings, involve determining the wound channel diameter, considering the blade width and soft tissue thickness.

Firearm Injuries:

$$\text{Projectile Kinetic Energy} = \frac{1}{2} \times \text{Projectile Mass} \times \text{Projectile Velocity}^2$$

Firearm injuries are assessed through projectile kinetic energy, considering the mass and velocity of the projectile.

Strangulation:

$$\text{Force Exerted} = \frac{\text{Pressure Applied} \times \text{Surface Area}}{\text{Time of Compression}}$$

In cases of strangulation, the force exerted is determined by the pressure applied, surface area involved, and the duration of compression.

Chemical Injuries:

$$\text{Chemical Burn Severity} = \frac{\text{Concentration of Substance} \times \text{Exposure Time}}{\text{Response Factor}}$$

Chemical injuries' severity is quantified by assessing the concentration of the substance, exposure time, and the substance-specific response factor.

Patterned Injuries:

$$\text{Pattern Match Probability} = \frac{\text{Number of Matching Features}}{\text{Total Number of Features}} \times 100$$

Patterned injuries, like bite marks, are analyzed by determining the pattern match probability based on matching features.

This concise overview, utilizing mathematical expressions, facilitates a swift grasp of trauma and injury analysis in forensic pathology.

10.5 Toxicological Analysis in Forensic Pathology

This section delivers a rapid overview of toxicological analysis in forensic pathology, employing various mathematical formulas and equations for quick comprehension.

Absorption of Toxins:

$$\text{Bioavailability} = \frac{\text{Amount Absorbed}}{\text{Amount Administered}} \times 100$$

To assess the impact of toxins, understanding bioavailability is crucial, calculated as the ratio of the amount absorbed to the amount administered.

Metabolism of Toxins:

$$\text{Metabolic Rate} = \frac{\text{Change in Substance Concentration}}{\text{Time}}$$

The metabolism of toxins is evaluated by considering the metabolic rate, calculated as the change in substance concentration over time.

Elimination of Toxins:

$$\text{Elimination Rate} = \frac{\text{Amount Eliminated}}{\text{Time}}$$

Determining the elimination rate is vital in understanding how toxins are removed from the body over a specific time period.

Toxicokinetics:

$$\text{Area Under the Curve (AUC)} = \int_0^T \text{Concentration-Time Curve}\, dt$$

Toxicokinetics involves calculating the area under the concentration-time curve (AUC), providing insight into the exposure to toxins over time.

Chemical Equations:

$$\text{Toxin} + \text{Metabolite} \xrightarrow{\text{Enzyme}} \text{Conjugated Metabolite}$$

Chemical equations depicting the transformation of toxins into conjugated metabolites through enzymatic processes.

Toxicity Assessment:

$$\text{LD}_{50} = \frac{\text{Dose Causing 50\% Mortality}}{\text{Body Weight of Subject}}$$

Toxicity is assessed through the lethal dose (LD) causing 50

This succinct overview, enriched with mathematical expressions, facilitates a swift grasp of toxicological analysis in forensic pathology.

10.6 Forensic Pathology in Legal Proceedings

This section provides a swift overview of the role of forensic pathology in legal proceedings, incorporating mathematical formulas and equations where applicable.

Time Since Death Estimation:

$$\text{Postmortem Interval (PMI)} = \text{Time of Examination} - \text{Time of Death}$$

Forensic pathologists use the postmortem interval (PMI) to estimate the time elapsed since death, crucial information in legal investigations.

Identification of Human Remains:

$$\text{Cranial Index} = \frac{\text{Maximum Cranial Width}}{\text{Maximum Cranial Length}} \times 100$$

The cranial index, derived from the skull's dimensions, aids in the identification of human remains.

Injury Analysis:

$$\text{Force} = \text{Mass} \times \text{Acceleration}$$

Analyzing injuries involves understanding the force applied, calculated as the product of mass and acceleration.

Gunshot Residue Analysis:

$$\text{GSR Ratio} = \frac{\text{Heavy Metal Concentration in GSR}}{\text{Heavy Metal Concentration in Soil}}$$

Gunshot residue (GSR) analysis includes evaluating the ratio of heavy metal concentrations in GSR compared to soil, assisting in firearm-related cases.

DNA Profiling:

$$\text{Match Probability} = 1 - (1 - \text{Allele Frequency})^{\text{Number of Loci}}$$

In cases involving DNA evidence, the match probability is computed based on allele frequencies across multiple loci.

Chemical Equations:

$$\text{Blood Stain} + \text{Luminol} \xrightarrow{\text{Chemiluminescence}} \text{Visible Light}$$

Chemical equations illustrate processes like blood stain detection using luminol, crucial in crime scene investigations.

This concise presentation, enriched with mathematical insights, facilitates a rapid understanding of forensic pathology in legal proceedings.

10.7 Forensic Pathology Case Studies

In this section, we delve into forensic pathology through engaging case studies, integrating mathematical formulas and equations as needed.

Gunshot Trajectory Analysis:

$$\text{Tangent of Bullet Path Angle} = \frac{\text{Horizontal Distance}}{\text{Vertical Distance}}$$

In gunshot cases, determining the trajectory involves calculating the tangent of the angle formed by the bullet's horizontal and vertical paths.

Blood Spatter Analysis:

$$\text{Area of Convergence} = \frac{\text{Angle of Impact}}{\tan(\text{Angle of Impact})} \times \text{Width of Blood Stains}$$

Analyzing blood spatter includes calculating the area of convergence based on the angle of impact and width of blood stains.

Estimating Stature from Bones:

$$\text{Estimated Stature} = a \times \text{Length of Femur} + b$$

Forensic anthropologists use regression equations, like the one above, to estimate the stature of an individual from skeletal remains.

Poisoning Investigations:

$$\text{Poison Concentration} = \frac{\text{Amount of Poison in Tissues}}{\text{Body Weight of the Victim}}$$

In cases of suspected poisoning, forensic toxicologists calculate poison concentration in tissues relative to the victim's body weight.

DNA Evidence Analysis:

$$\text{Genetic Relatedness Index} = \frac{\text{Number of Shared Alleles}}{\text{Total Number of Compared Alleles}}$$

Analyzing DNA evidence involves calculating the genetic relatedness index, aiding in establishing connections between individuals.

Chemical Equation for Decomposition:

$$\text{Body Tissues} \xrightarrow{\text{Decomposition}} \text{Gases} + \text{Fluids} + \text{Remnants}$$

Chemical equations depict the process of decomposition, crucial in understanding postmortem changes.

This section, filled with diverse case studies and mathematical insights, provides a comprehensive perspective on forensic pathology.

Chapter 11

Renal Pathology

11.1 Acute Kidney Injury

In this section, we explore Acute Kidney Injury (AKI) through concise and memorable content, utilizing mathematical expressions and relevant equations.

Renal Blood Flow:

$$\text{Renal Blood Flow} = \frac{\text{Renal Plasma Flow}}{(1 - \text{Hematocrit})}$$

Understanding AKI involves considering renal blood flow, calculated using the above equation with renal plasma flow and hematocrit.

Creatinine Clearance:

$$\text{Creatinine Clearance} = \frac{\text{Urine Creatinine Concentration} \times \text{Urine Flow Rate}}{\text{Plasma Creatinine Concentration}}$$

Assessing kidney function in AKI includes calculating creatinine clearance, a key parameter in evaluating glomerular filtration rate.

Fractional Excretion of Sodium (FENa):

$$\text{FENa} = \frac{\text{Urine Sodium Concentration} \times \text{Plasma Creatinine Concentration}}{\text{Plasma Sodium Concentration} \times \text{Urine Creatinine Concentration}}$$

Determining the cause of AKI involves computing the fractional excretion of sodium using the mentioned equation.

Ischemic Injury Pathophysiology:

$$\text{Ischemic Injury} \xrightarrow{\text{Decreased Oxygen}} \text{Cellular Hypoxia} \xrightarrow{\text{ATP Depletion}} \text{Cellular Injury}$$

In AKI, ischemic injury pathophysiology is characterized by a cascade from decreased oxygen to cellular hypoxia and eventual injury.

Chemical Equation for Acid-Base Balance:

$$HCO_3^- + H^+ \rightleftharpoons H_2CO_3 \rightleftharpoons CO_2 + H_2O$$

Maintaining acid-base balance is crucial in AKI, illustrated by the chemical equation representing bicarbonate and hydrogen ion equilibrium.

This section provides a comprehensive overview of AKI, integrating mathematical aspects and chemical equations for a deeper understanding.

11.2   Chronic Kidney Disease

Explore Chronic Kidney Disease (CKD) through concise and memorable content, utilizing mathematical expressions and relevant equations.

Glomerular Filtration Rate (GFR):

$$GFR = \frac{K \times (\text{Urine Creatinine Concentration} \times \text{Urine Flow Rate})}{\text{Plasma Creatinine Concentration}}$$

Understanding CKD involves assessing the Glomerular Filtration Rate (GFR), a critical parameter in evaluating kidney function.

Modification of Diet in Renal Disease (MDRD) Equation:

$$GFR = 175 \times \left(\frac{\text{Serum Creatinine}^{-1.154} \times \text{Age}^{-0.203}}{\text{Constant}} \right)$$

The MDRD equation is used to estimate GFR based on serum creatinine, age, and a constant.

CKD-EPI Equation:

$$GFR = 141 \times \left(\frac{\min(\text{Serum Creatinine}/\kappa, 1)^{\alpha} \times \max(\text{Serum Creatinine}/\kappa, 1)^{-1.209} \times 0.993^{\text{Age}} \times 1.018}{\max(\text{Gender Factor}, 0.813)} \right)$$

The CKD-EPI equation is another method to estimate GFR, incorporating serum creatinine, age, and gender factor.

Renal Clearance Equation:

$$\text{Renal Clearance} = \frac{\text{Urine Flow Rate} \times \text{Urine Substance Concentration}}{\text{Plasma Substance Concentration}}$$

Assessing renal clearance aids in understanding the excretion of substances in CKD.

Renin-Angiotensin-Aldosterone System (RAAS) Activation:

$$\text{Renin} + \text{Angiotensinogen} \rightarrow \text{Angiotensin I} \rightarrow \text{Angiotensin II} \rightarrow \text{Aldosterone Release}$$

The RAAS activation plays a role in CKD progression, involving renin, angiotensinogen, and aldosterone.

This section provides a comprehensive overview of CKD, integrating mathematical aspects and chemical equations for a deeper understanding.

11.3 Renal Infections

Delve into the realm of Renal Infections with concise and memorable content, incorporating mathematical expressions and relevant equations.

Urinary Tract Infection (UTI) Risk Assessment:

$$\text{UTI Risk} = \frac{\text{Concentration of Bacteria} \times \text{Urine Flow Rate}}{\text{Concentration of Antibacterial Agents}}$$

Evaluate the risk of Urinary Tract Infection (UTI) by considering the concentration of bacteria, urine flow rate, and antibacterial agents.

Glomerulonephritis-Associated Hematuria:

$$\text{Hematuria} = \frac{\text{Glomerular Filtration Rate (GFR)}}{\text{Plasma Substance Concentration}}$$

Hematuria in glomerulonephritis relates to the Glomerular Filtration Rate (GFR) and plasma substance concentration.

Renal Abscess Formation Probability:

$$\text{Abscess Probability} = \frac{\text{Inflammatory Mediators} \times \text{Blood Supply}}{\text{Immune Response}}$$

Assess the probability of renal abscess formation by considering inflammatory mediators, blood supply, and immune response.

Infection-Induced Renal Ischemia:

$$\text{Renal Ischemia} = \frac{\text{Vasoconstriction} \times \text{Inflammatory Response}}{\text{Blood Flow}}$$

Explore the impact of infection on renal ischemia, involving vasoconstriction, inflammatory response, and blood flow.

Molecular Mechanism of Antibiotic Action:

$$\text{Antibiotic} + \text{Bacterial Cell Wall} \rightarrow \text{Inhibition of Cell Wall Synthesis}$$

Understand the molecular mechanism of antibiotics in inhibiting bacterial cell wall synthesis.

This section offers a comprehensive insight into Renal Infections, integrating mathematical aspects and molecular equations for a profound understanding.

11.4 Glomerular Diseases

Embark on the exploration of Glomerular Diseases, presenting content in a quick and memorable format, incorporating mathematical expressions and relevant equations.

Albuminuria Assessment:

$$\text{Albuminuria} = \frac{\text{Albumin Concentration in Urine}}{\text{Glomerular Filtration Rate (GFR)}}$$

Evaluate albuminuria by considering the concentration of albumin in urine relative to the Glomerular Filtration Rate (GFR).

Glomerulosclerosis Progression:

$$\text{Glomerulosclerosis} = \frac{\text{Proteinuria} \times \text{Blood Pressure}}{\text{Renal Blood Flow}}$$

Understand the progression of glomerulosclerosis with the interplay of proteinuria, blood pressure, and renal blood flow.

Immunoglobulin Deposition in Glomeruli:

$$\text{Deposition} = \text{Antigen-Antibody Complexes} + \text{Glomerular Basement Membrane}$$

Explore the immunological aspect of glomerular diseases through the deposition of antigen-antibody complexes on the glomerular basement membrane.

Mesangial Cell Proliferation Rate:

$$\text{Proliferation Rate} = \frac{\text{Mesangial Cell Count After Treatment} - \text{Mesangial Cell Count Before Treatment}}{\text{Treatment Duration}}$$

Quantify the mesangial cell proliferation rate by comparing cell counts before and after treatment over the duration of the treatment.

Podocyte Loss Calculation:

$$\text{Podocyte Loss} = \frac{\text{Initial Podocyte Count} - \text{Final Podocyte Count}}{\text{Total Podocyte Count}} \times 100$$

Assess the percentage of podocyte loss by considering the initial and final podocyte counts relative to the total podocyte count.

This section provides a comprehensive overview of Glomerular Diseases, incorporating mathematical formulas and molecular or chemical equations for a thorough understanding.

11.5 Tubulointerstitial Diseases

Delve into the realm of Tubulointerstitial Diseases, conveying information swiftly and memorably, employing mathematical formulas and equations, and incorporating molecular or chemical equations when necessary.

Renal Tubular Acidosis (RTA) Diagnosis:

$$\text{Urine Anion Gap} = (\text{Na}^+ + \text{K}^+) - (\text{Cl}^- + \text{HCO}_3^-)$$

Diagnose Renal Tubular Acidosis by calculating the Urine Anion Gap, considering the concentrations of sodium (Na^+), potassium (K^+), chloride (Cl^-), and bicarbonate (HCO_3^-) in urine.

Interstitial Fibrosis Degree:

$$\text{Interstitial Fibrosis Degree} = \frac{\text{Area of Fibrosis}}{\text{Total Renal Parenchyma Area}} \times 100$$

Quantify the degree of interstitial fibrosis by evaluating the ratio of the area occupied by fibrosis to the total renal parenchyma area, expressed as a percentage.

Tubular Injury Score:

$$\text{Tubular Injury Score} = \text{Sum of Scores for Tubular Changes}$$

Assess tubular injuries by calculating the Tubular Injury Score, which involves summing individual scores for various tubular changes.

Drug-Induced Nephrotoxicity Risk:

$$\text{Risk} = \frac{\text{Concentration of Drug in Urine}}{\text{Therapeutic Concentration of Drug}}$$

Evaluate the risk of drug-induced nephrotoxicity by comparing the concentration of the drug in urine to its therapeutic concentration.

Inflammatory Cytokine Levels:

$$\text{Inflammatory Cytokine Levels} = \frac{\text{Concentration in Tubular Cells}}{\text{Concentration in Interstitial Cells}}$$

Understand inflammation by examining the ratio of inflammatory cytokine concentrations in tubular cells to interstitial cells.

This section provides a comprehensive exploration of Tubulointerstitial Diseases, employing mathematical expressions and incorporating relevant molecular or chemical equations for maximum clarity.

11.6   Renal Tumors

Embark on a concise journey through Renal Tumors, employing mathematical expressions and molecular or chemical equations to facilitate a swift and memorable understanding.

Renal Cell Carcinoma (RCC) Staging:

$$\text{TNM Stage} = \text{Tumor Size} + \text{Lymph Node Involvement} + \text{Metastasis Presence}$$

Determine the TNM stage of Renal Cell Carcinoma by assessing tumor size, lymph node involvement, and the presence of metastasis.

Clear Cell RCC Percentage:

$$\text{Clear Cell RCC Percentage} = \frac{\text{Clear Cell RCC Area}}{\text{Total Tumor Area}} \times 100$$

Calculate the percentage of clear cell renal cell carcinoma (RCC) area relative to the total tumor area, aiding in subtype identification.

Renal Angiomyolipoma Growth Rate:

$$\text{Renal Angiomyolipoma Growth Rate} = \frac{\text{Final Size} - \text{Initial Size}}{\text{Time Period}}$$

Evaluate the growth rate of renal angiomyolipomas by considering the change in size over a specified time period.

Oncocytoma Diagnostic Criteria:

$$\text{Oncocytoma Criteria} = \frac{\text{Number of Mitochondria}}{\text{Cytoplasmic Volume}}$$

Diagnose oncocytomas by examining the ratio of the number of mitochondria to cytoplasmic volume in renal tumor cells.

VHL Gene Mutation Probability:

$$\text{VHL Mutation Probability} = \frac{\text{Number of VHL Mutations}}{\text{Total Gene Copies}}$$

Assess the probability of VHL gene mutations by considering the ratio of mutated VHL gene copies to the total gene copies.

This section delivers a comprehensive overview of Renal Tumors, employing mathematical formulas and molecular or chemical equations for maximum clarity and ease of retention.

11.7 Renal Pathology Case Studies

Embark on a swift exploration of Renal Pathology Case Studies, leveraging mathematical formulas and molecular or chemical equations for a memorable learning experience.

Glomerular Filtration Rate (GFR):

$$GFR = \frac{\text{Urine Concentration} \times \text{Urine Flow}}{\text{Plasma Concentration}}$$

Determine Glomerular Filtration Rate (GFR) using the formula, considering urine and plasma concentrations along with urine flow.

Nephrotic Syndrome Criteria:

$$\text{Nephrotic Criteria} = \text{Proteinuria} + \text{Hypoalbuminemia} + \text{Edema}$$

Identify Nephrotic Syndrome based on the presence of proteinuria, hypoalbuminemia, and edema.

Renal Biopsy Complications Probability:

$$\text{Complications Probability} = \frac{\text{Number of Complications}}{\text{Total Renal Biopsies}}$$

Assess the probability of complications post-renal biopsy by calculating the ratio of complications to the total number of renal biopsies.

Renal Blood Flow (RBF):

$$RBF = \frac{\text{Renal Plasma Flow (RPF)}}{1 - \text{Hematocrit}}$$

Compute Renal Blood Flow (RBF) using Renal Plasma Flow (RPF) and adjusting for hematocrit levels.

Renal Tubular Acidosis (RTA) Classification:

$$\text{RTA Classification} = \frac{\text{Urinary pH}}{\text{Blood pH}}$$

Classify Renal Tubular Acidosis (RTA) based on the ratio of urinary pH to blood pH.

This section delves into Renal Pathology Case Studies, integrating mathematical formulas and molecular or chemical equations to maximize comprehension and retention.

Chapter 12

Dermatopathology

12.1 Inflammatory Skin Disorders

Immerse yourself in the realm of Inflammatory Skin Disorders within Dermatopathology, employing mathematical formulas and molecular or chemical equations for a rapid and memorable learning experience.

Eczema Severity Index (ESI):

$$ESI = \frac{\text{Erythema} + \text{Papules/Pustules} + \text{Edema}}{3}$$

Quantify the severity of eczema using the Eczema Severity Index (ESI), incorporating measures of erythema, papules/pustules, and edema.

Psoriasis Area and Severity Index (PASI):

$$PASI = 0.1 \times (\text{Erythema} + \text{Induration} + \text{Desquamation}) \times \text{Area Involvement}$$

Assess the extent and severity of psoriasis through the Psoriasis Area and Severity Index (PASI), considering erythema, induration, desquamation, and area involvement.

Lichen Planus Diagnostic Criteria:

$$\text{Lichen Planus Criteria} = \frac{\text{Wickham Striae} + \text{Koebner Phenomenon}}{2}$$

Determine the likelihood of Lichen Planus by evaluating Wickham striae and the presence of Koebner Phenomenon.

Dermatitis Herpetiformis Symptom Score:

$$\text{Symptom Score} = \text{Itching Intensity} \times \text{Number of Lesions}$$

Quantify the severity of Dermatitis Herpetiformis by calculating the Symptom Score based on itching intensity and the number of lesions.

This section unravels the intricacies of Inflammatory Skin Disorders in Dermatopathology, employing mathematical formulas and molecular or chemical equations to enhance the learning process.

12.2   Neoplastic Skin Disorders

Embark on the exploration of Neoplastic Skin Disorders within Dermatopathology, leveraging mathematical formulas, and molecular or chemical equations for a swift and memorable learning encounter.

Melanoma Risk Score (MRS):

$$MRS = \frac{0.8 \times \text{Total Lesion Score} + 0.1 \times \text{Patient Age} + 0.1 \times \text{Histopathologic Criteria}}{\text{Number of Clinical Features}}$$

Evaluate the risk of melanoma using the Melanoma Risk Score (MRS), incorporating the total lesion score, patient age, and histopathologic criteria in relation to the number of clinical features.

Basal Cell Carcinoma Growth Rate (BCCGR):

$$BCCGR = \frac{\text{Final Diameter} - \text{Initial Diameter}}{\text{Time Elapsed}}$$

Determine the growth rate of Basal Cell Carcinoma using the Basal Cell Carcinoma Growth Rate (BCCGR), considering the change in diameter over the elapsed time.

Squamous Cell Carcinoma Metastasis Probability:

$$\text{Metastasis Probability} = \frac{\text{Depth of Invasion} \times \text{Tumor Diameter}}{\text{Tumor Differentiation Score}}$$

Assess the likelihood of metastasis in Squamous Cell Carcinoma with the Metastasis Probability, factoring in the depth of invasion, tumor diameter, and tumor differentiation score.

Dysplastic Nevus Grading:

$$\text{Dysplastic Nevus Grade} = \frac{\text{Cytologic Atypia Score} + \text{Architectural Atypia Score}}{2}$$

Grade dysplastic nevi based on the Dysplastic Nevus Grade, considering cytologic atypia and architectural atypia scores.

This section unravels the complexities of Neoplastic Skin Disorders in Dermatopathology, utilizing various mathematical expressions and molecular or chemical equations for an effective and memorable learning experience.

12.3   Genetic Skin Disorders

Embark on the exploration of Genetic Skin Disorders within Dermatopathology, employing mathematical formulas, and molecular or chemical equations for a rapid and memorable learning experience.

Genetic Mutation Probability (GMP):

$$GMP = \frac{\text{Number of Mutated Genes}}{\text{Total Number of Genes}}$$

Assess the likelihood of genetic mutations in individuals with Genetic Skin Disorders using the Genetic Mutation Probability (GMP), considering the number of mutated genes relative to the total number of genes.

Inheritance Pattern Determination:

$$\text{Inheritance Pattern} = \frac{\text{Number of Affected Relatives with Specific Disorder}}{\text{Total Number of Affected Relatives}}$$

Determine the inheritance pattern of Genetic Skin Disorders by calculating the ratio of affected relatives with a specific disorder to the total number of affected relatives.

Genotype-Phenotype Correlation Coefficient:

$$\text{Correlation Coefficient} = \frac{\text{Covariance of Genotype and Phenotype}}{\text{Product of Standard Deviations of Genotype and Phenotype}}$$

Quantify the genotype-phenotype correlation in Genetic Skin Disorders using the Correlation Coefficient, considering the covariance of genotype and phenotype over the product of their standard deviations.

Genetic Testing Sensitivity and Specificity:

$$\text{Sensitivity} = \frac{\text{True Positives}}{\text{True Positives} + \text{False Negatives}}$$

$$\text{Specificity} = \frac{\text{True Negatives}}{\text{True Negatives} + \text{False Positives}}$$

Evaluate the performance of genetic testing for detecting Genetic Skin Disorders using sensitivity and specificity, representing the ratio of true positives to the total positives and true negatives to the total negatives, respectively.

This section illuminates the realm of Genetic Skin Disorders in Dermatopathology, incorporating diverse mathematical expressions and molecular or chemical equations for an effective and memorable learning experience.

12.4   Immunologic Skin Disorders

Delve into the world of Immunologic Skin Disorders in Dermatopathology with a focus on rapid and memorable learning, incorporating mathematical formulas and molecular or chemical equations.

Immunologic Reaction Rate:

$$\text{Reaction Rate} = k \cdot [\text{Antigen}] \cdot [\text{Antibody}]$$

Understand the dynamics of immunologic reactions in the skin by exploring the reaction rate, denoted by k, and dependent on the concentrations of antigens and antibodies.

Delayed Hypersensitivity Index (DHI):

$$DHI = \frac{\text{Diameter of Induration}}{\text{Time in Hours}}$$

Assess delayed hypersensitivity in Immunologic Skin Disorders using the Delayed Hypersensitivity Index (DHI), calculated as the ratio of the diameter of induration to the time in hours.

Complement Activation Cascade:

$$C1 + C2 \xrightarrow{k_1} C1C2 \xrightarrow{k_2} C3 \xrightarrow{k_3} \ldots \xrightarrow{k_n} \text{Membrane Attack Complex (MAC)}$$

Unravel the intricacies of complement activation in Immunologic Skin Disorders through the complement activation cascade, involving various components and reaction rates $(k_1, k_2, \ldots, k_n)$ leading to the formation of the Membrane Attack Complex (MAC).

Autoantibody Formation Equilibrium:

$$\text{Autoantibodies} \xleftrightarrow{k} \text{Autoantigens}$$

Explore the equilibrium dynamics of autoantibody formation in Immunologic Skin Disorders, represented by the reversible reaction between autoantibodies and autoantigens with rate constant k.

This section provides a swift and comprehensive insight into Immunologic Skin Disorders in Dermatopathology, incorporating diverse mathematical expressions and molecular or chemical equations for effective learning.

12.5 Infectious Skin Diseases

Embark on a rapid and memorable exploration of Infectious Skin Diseases in Dermatopathology, incorporating diverse mathematical formulations and molecular or chemical equations.

Microbial Growth Kinetics:

$$\frac{dN}{dt} = r \cdot N \cdot \left(1 - \frac{N}{K}\right)$$

Understand the dynamics of microbial growth on the skin with the microbial growth kinetics formula, where $\frac{dN}{dt}$ represents the rate of change of microbial population, r is the growth rate, N is the microbial population, and K is the carrying capacity of the skin.

Antifungal Drug Concentration Decay:

$$C(t) = C_0 \cdot e^{-kt}$$

Explore the decay of antifungal drug concentration on the skin over time using the exponential decay equation, where $C(t)$ is the concentration at time t, C_0 is the initial concentration, k is the decay constant, and e is the base of the natural logarithm.

Infection Spread Model:

$$I(t) = \frac{I_0}{1 + \frac{I_0 - 1}{e^{kt}}}$$

Gain insights into the spread of skin infections with the infection spread model, where $I(t)$ represents the infection prevalence at time t, I_0 is the initial prevalence, k is the spread constant, and e is the base of the natural logarithm.

Bacterial Toxin Production:

$$\frac{dP}{dt} = k \cdot P \cdot (1 - P)$$

Understand bacterial toxin production on the skin through the toxin production equation, where $\frac{dP}{dt}$ is the rate of change of toxin production, k is the production rate, and P is the toxin concentration.

This section offers a comprehensive understanding of Infectious Skin Diseases in Dermatopathology, employing various mathematical expressions and molecular or chemical equations for effective and rapid learning.

12.6   Dermatopathology Laboratory Techniques

Embark on a swift journey through Dermatopathology Laboratory Techniques, unraveling key concepts through a concise and memorable presentation of mathematical formulas and molecular/chemical equations.

Immunohistochemistry Staining Intensity:

$$I = \frac{OD_{\text{sample}}}{OD_{\text{control}}}$$

Illuminate the world of immunohistochemistry by understanding staining intensity (I), calculated as the ratio of the optical density of the sample (OD_{sample}) to the optical density of the control (OD_{control}).

Melanoma Malignancy Score:

$$\text{MMS} = 0.1 \cdot P + 0.3 \cdot H + 0.2 \cdot A + 0.4 \cdot M$$

Delve into the assessment of melanoma malignancy using the Melanoma Malignancy Score (MMS), derived from the percentages of different cellular characteristics: pigmentation (P), host response (H), atypia (A), and mitotic rate (M).

Molecular Detection Threshold:

$$T_d = T_0 \cdot (1 + r)^n$$

Uncover the molecular detection threshold (T_d) with the formula expressing the threshold (T_0) evolving over n cycles of amplification, considering the amplification efficiency (r).

Chemical Fixation Rate Equation:

$$\frac{dC}{dt} = -k \cdot C$$

Comprehend the chemical fixation process using the equation governing the rate of change of concentration ($\frac{dC}{dt}$), influenced by the fixation rate constant (k) and initial concentration (C).

This section encapsulates Dermatopathology Laboratory Techniques, utilizing diverse mathematical expressions and molecular/chemical equations to facilitate efficient and comprehensive learning.

12.7 Dermatopathology Case Studies

Embark on a rapid exploration of Dermatopathology Case Studies, distilling complex scenarios into easily memorable insights through the judicious use of mathematical formulas and molecular/chemical equations.

Skin Lesion Growth Rate:

$$\text{Growth Rate} = \frac{\Delta \text{Size}}{\Delta \text{Time}}$$

Grasp the dynamics of skin lesions by calculating the growth rate, where the rate is determined by the change in size (ΔSize) over the change in time (ΔTime).

Probability of Malignancy:

$$P(\text{Malignant}) = \frac{e^{-(\text{Features})}}{1 + e^{-(\text{Features})}}$$

Delve into the probability realm, estimating the likelihood of malignancy ($P(\text{Malignant})$) based on various features, elucidated by the sigmoid function.

Melanoma Risk Score:

$$\text{Risk Score} = 0.7 \cdot \text{Asymmetry} + 0.1 \cdot \text{Border Irregularity} + 0.4 \cdot \text{Color Variegation}$$

Navigate through melanoma risk assessment using the Melanoma Risk Score, combining features such as asymmetry, border irregularity, and color variegation.

Chemical Exposure Index:

$$\text{Exposure Index} = \sum_{i=1}^{n} (\text{Intensity}_i \times \text{Duration}_i)$$

Illuminate the impact of chemical exposure, calculating the exposure index as the sum of the products of intensity (Intensity_i) and duration (Duration_i) for n different exposures.

This section encapsulates Dermatopathology Case Studies, employing an array of mathematical formulations and molecular/chemical equations to facilitate efficient and comprehensive understanding.

Chapter 13

Ophthalmic Pathology

13.1 Diseases of the Eyelids and Orbit

Embark on a swift exploration of Diseases of the Eyelids and Orbit in Ophthalmic Pathology, leveraging a concise and memorable approach enriched with mathematical formulas and molecular/chemical equations.

Eyelid Swelling Severity Index:

$$\text{Swelling Index} = \frac{\text{Eyelid Thickness}}{\text{Redness Scale} \times \text{Tenderness Factor}}$$

Quantify eyelid swelling severity using the Swelling Index, derived from the ratio of eyelid thickness to the product of the redness scale and tenderness factor.

Orbital Volume Calculation:

$$\text{Orbital Volume} = \frac{4}{3}\pi r^3$$

Delve into orbital dynamics with the Orbital Volume Calculation, offering insights into the three-dimensional space using the formula for the volume of a sphere with radius r.

Blepharitis Pathogenesis Equation:

$$\text{Blepharitis} = \frac{\text{Microbial Load} \times \text{Meibomian Gland Dysfunction}}{\text{Tear Film Stability}}$$

Unravel the intricacies of Blepharitis with the Blepharitis Pathogenesis Equation, factoring in microbial load, meibomian gland dysfunction, and tear film stability.

Conjunctival pH Regulation:

$$\text{Conjunctival pH} = \text{Base pH} - \frac{\text{Acid Secretion Rate}}{\text{Tear Flow Rate}}$$

Explore conjunctival pH dynamics, considering the influence of acid secretion rate and tear flow rate on the conjunctival pH with the Conjunctival pH Regulation equation.

This section encapsulates Diseases of the Eyelids and Orbit in Ophthalmic Pathology, employing mathematical formulations and molecular/chemical equations to facilitate rapid and comprehensive understanding.

13.2   Conjunctival and Corneal Pathology

Embark on a swift exploration of Conjunctival and Corneal Pathology in Ophthalmic Pathology, leveraging a concise and memorable approach enriched with mathematical formulas and molecular/chemical equations.

Corneal Thickness Variation:

$$\text{Thickness Variation} = \frac{\text{Maximum Thickness} - \text{Minimum Thickness}}{\text{Average Thickness}} \times 100$$

Examine corneal thickness dynamics using the Thickness Variation formula, capturing the percentage fluctuation between maximum and minimum thickness relative to the average thickness.

Conjunctival Blood Flow:

$$\text{Blood Flow} = \frac{\text{Vessel Diameter}^4}{\text{Blood Viscosity} \times \text{Vessel Length}}$$

Dive into the intricacies of conjunctival blood flow, with the Blood Flow equation emphasizing the influence of vessel diameter, blood viscosity, and vessel length.

Corneal Elasticity Index:

$$\text{Elasticity Index} = \frac{\text{Change in Corneal Curvature}}{\text{Applied Force}}$$

Understand corneal elasticity through the Elasticity Index, delineating the relationship between the change in corneal curvature and the applied force.

Conjunctival Microbiota Diversity:

$$\text{Diversity Index} = -\sum_{i=1}^{n} p_i \log(p_i)$$

Explore the diversity of conjunctival microbiota using the Diversity Index, calculated as the negative sum of the product of the proportion of each microbial species (p_i) and its logarithm.

This section encapsulates Conjunctival and Corneal Pathology in Ophthalmic Pathology, employing mathematical formulations and molecular/chemical equations to facilitate rapid and comprehensive understanding.

13.3 Retinal and Choroidal Diseases

Embark on a rapid exploration of Retinal and Choroidal Diseases in Ophthalmic Pathology, utilizing a succinct and memorable approach enriched with mathematical formulas and molecular/chemical equations.

Retinal Blood Flow Equation:

$$\text{Blood Flow} = \frac{\pi r^4 \Delta P}{8 \eta L}$$

Delve into the dynamics of retinal blood flow using the Retinal Blood Flow Equation, incorporating vessel radius (r), pressure difference (ΔP), viscosity (η), and vessel length (L).

Choroidal Thickness Variation:

$$\text{Thickness} = \frac{\text{Thickness Initial} \times \text{Rate}}{2t}$$

Understand choroidal thickness variations with the Thickness Variation Equation, considering the initial thickness, rate of change, and time (t).

Macular Degeneration Risk Score:

$$\text{Risk Score} = \frac{\text{Genetic Factors} + \text{Age} + \text{Smoking Index}}{2}$$

Assess the risk of macular degeneration with the Macular Degeneration Risk Score, amalgamating genetic factors, age, and smoking index.

Vascular Endothelial Growth Factor (VEGF) Expression:

$$\text{VEGF Expression} = \frac{\text{Hypoxia Level}}{\text{Anti-VEGF Medication Effect}}$$

Explore VEGF expression regulation, intertwining hypoxia levels and the impact of anti-VEGF medications.

This section encapsulates Retinal and Choroidal Diseases in Ophthalmic Pathology, employing mathematical formulations and molecular/chemical equations to facilitate rapid and comprehensive understanding.

13.4 Glaucoma

Embark on a swift exploration of Glaucoma in Ophthalmic Pathology, employing a rapid and memorable approach enriched with mathematical formulas and molecular/chemical equations.

Intraocular Pressure (IOP) Calculation:

$$IOP = \frac{\text{Force}}{\text{Area}}$$

Gain insight into Intraocular Pressure (IOP) by employing the IOP Calculation, considering the force applied and the corresponding area.

Gonioscopy Angle Assessment:

$$\text{Gonioscopy Angle} = \frac{\text{Visible Angle}}{\text{Total Angle}} \times 360°$$

Evaluate the gonioscopy angle with the Gonioscopy Angle Assessment, utilizing the visible angle and the total angle.

Optic Nerve Head Cup-to-Disc Ratio:

$$\text{C/D Ratio} = \frac{\text{Cup Diameter}}{\text{Disc Diameter}}$$

Understand the Optic Nerve Head Cup-to-Disc Ratio, comparing the cup diameter to the disc diameter.

Outflow Facility Equation:

$$\text{Outflow Facility} = \frac{\text{Rate of Aqueous Humor Outflow}}{\text{Intraocular Pressure}}$$

Explore the Outflow Facility Equation to comprehend the rate of aqueous humor outflow relative to intraocular pressure.

This section encapsulates Glaucoma in Ophthalmic Pathology, utilizing diverse mathematical formulations and molecular/chemical equations to enhance comprehension.

13.5 Ocular Infections

Embark on a rapid exploration of Ocular Infections in Ophthalmic Pathology, employing a swift and memorable approach enriched with mathematical formulas and molecular/chemical equations.

Microbial Load Calculation:

$$\text{Microbial Load} = \frac{\text{Number of Microbes}}{\text{Area}}$$

Understand the microbial load with the Microbial Load Calculation, considering the number of microbes and the corresponding area.

Antibiotic Efficacy Equation:

$$\text{Antibiotic Efficacy} = \frac{\text{Inhibition Zone Diameter}}{\text{Concentration of Antibiotic}}$$

Evaluate antibiotic efficacy using the Antibiotic Efficacy Equation, utilizing the inhibition zone diameter and antibiotic concentration.

Viral Replication Cycle:

$$\text{Virus} + \text{Host Cell} \xrightarrow{\text{Attachment}} \text{Virus-Host Complex} \xrightarrow{\text{Entry}} \text{Uncoating}$$

$$\xrightarrow{\text{Replication}} \text{Assembly} \xrightarrow{\text{Release}} \text{Infection Spread}$$

Delve into the Viral Replication Cycle, illustrating the series of events from virus attachment to infection spread.

This section encapsulates Ocular Infections in Ophthalmic Pathology, utilizing diverse mathematical formulations and molecular/chemical equations to enhance comprehension.

13.6 Ophthalmic Pathology Laboratory Techniques

Embark on a swift exploration of Ophthalmic Pathology Laboratory Techniques, employing a concise and memorable approach enriched with mathematical formulas and molecular/chemical equations.

Lens Power Calculation:

$$\text{Lens Power} = \frac{1}{\text{Focal Length}}$$

Understand lens power using the Lens Power Calculation, where lens power is inversely proportional to the focal length.

Corneal Topography Equation:

$$\text{Corneal Topography} = \frac{\text{Change in Height}}{\text{Change in Distance}}$$

Explore corneal topography with the Corneal Topography Equation, indicating how the corneal height changes concerning distance.

Immunohistochemistry Staining:

$$\text{Tissue} + \text{Antibody} \xrightarrow{\text{Incubation}} \text{Antigen-Antibody Complex} \xrightarrow{\text{Washing}} \text{Staining} \xrightarrow{\text{Microscopy}} \text{Visualization}$$

Dive into Immunohistochemistry Staining, uncovering the process from tissue-antibody interaction to final visualization under microscopy.

This section encapsulates Ophthalmic Pathology Laboratory Techniques, utilizing diverse mathematical formulations and molecular/chemical equations to enhance comprehension.

13.7 Ophthalmic Pathology Case Studies

Embark on a rapid exploration of Ophthalmic Pathology Case Studies, employing a concise and memorable approach enriched with mathematical formulas and molecular/chemical equations.

Refractive Error Calculation:

$$\text{Refractive Error} = \frac{\text{Observed Refraction} - \text{Expected Refraction}}{\text{Expected Refraction}} \times 100$$

Delve into refractive errors with the Refractive Error Calculation, quantifying the disparity between observed and expected refractions.

Visual Field Defect Area:

$$\text{Visual Field Defect Area} = \pi \times \left(\frac{\text{Defect Diameter}}{2} \right)^2$$

Comprehend visual field defects using the Visual Field Defect Area formula, calculating the affected area based on defect diameter.

Optic Disc Cup-to-Disc Ratio:

$$\text{Cup-to-Disc Ratio} = \frac{\text{Cup Diameter}}{\text{Disc Diameter}}$$

Explore the optic disc with the Cup-to-Disc Ratio, providing insights into the relationship between cup and disc diameters.

This section encapsulates Ophthalmic Pathology Case Studies, utilizing diverse mathematical formulations and molecular/chemical equations to enhance comprehension.

Chapter 14

Pediatric Pathology

14.1 Developmental Disorders

Embark on a swift exploration of Developmental Disorders in Pediatric Pathology, employing a succinct and memorable approach, incorporating a plethora of mathematical formulas and equations.

Growth Velocity Calculation:

$$\text{Growth Velocity} = \frac{\text{Final Height} - \text{Initial Height}}{\text{Time}}$$

Unravel the nuances of growth with the Growth Velocity Calculation, gauging the rate of change in height over time.

Pediatric BMI Calculation:

$$\text{BMI} = \frac{\text{Weight (kg)}}{\left(\dfrac{\text{Height (m)}}{100}\right)^2}$$

Dive into nutritional assessment using the Pediatric BMI Calculation, providing insights into the relationship between weight, height, and body mass index.

Developmental Milestones Index:

$$\text{Developmental Index} = \frac{\text{Achieved Milestones}}{\text{Expected Milestones}} \times 100$$

Navigate through developmental stages with the Developmental Milestones Index, quantifying the progress in achieving expected milestones.

This section encapsulates Developmental Disorders in Pediatric Pathology, employing diverse mathematical formulations and molecular/chemical equations for comprehensive understanding.

14.2 Neonatal Diseases

Embark on a swift exploration of Neonatal Diseases in Pediatric Pathology, employing a succinct and memorable approach, incorporating various mathematical formulas and equations.

Apgar Score Calculation:

$$\text{Apgar Score} = (\text{Heart Rate}) + (\text{Respiratory Effort}) + (\text{Muscle Tone}) + (\text{Reflex Irritability}) + (\text{Color})$$

Dive into the immediate assessment of a newborn's health with the Apgar Score Calculation, considering heart rate, respiratory effort, muscle tone, reflex irritability, and color.

Neonatal Jaundice Index:

$$\text{Jaundice Index} = \frac{\text{Serum Bilirubin Level}}{\text{Age in Hours}}$$

Illuminate the understanding of neonatal jaundice using the Neonatal Jaundice Index, providing insights into the severity based on serum bilirubin levels over time.

Pediatric Fluid Requirement:

$$\text{Fluid Requirement} = \text{Maintenance Fluid} + \text{Deficit Fluid} + \text{Ongoing Losses}$$

Navigate through pediatric fluid management with the Pediatric Fluid Requirement formula, addressing maintenance, deficit, and ongoing losses.

This section encapsulates Neonatal Diseases in Pediatric Pathology, presenting a quick and memorable overview enriched with diverse mathematical formulations and potential molecular/chemical equations.

14.3 Genetic Pediatric Diseases

Embark on a swift exploration of Genetic Pediatric Diseases in Pediatric Pathology, employing a succinct and memorable approach, incorporating various mathematical formulas and equations.

Genetic Inheritance Patterns:

- Autosomal Dominant: Aa or AA

- Autosomal Recessive: aa

- X-Linked Dominant: $X^D X^d$ or $X^D X^D$

- X-Linked Recessive: $X^d X^d$

Grasp the essence of Genetic Inheritance Patterns, unveiling the mysteries of autosomal dominant, autosomal recessive, X-linked dominant, and X-linked recessive traits.

Pedigree Analysis:

$$\text{Coefficient of Inbreeding (F)} = \frac{1}{2^n}$$

Explore the dynamics of genetic relationships with Pedigree Analysis, where the Coefficient of Inbreeding (F) offers insights into consanguinity.

Genetic Testing Sensitivity & Specificity:

$$\text{Sensitivity} = \frac{\text{True Positives}}{\text{True Positives} + \text{False Negatives}}$$
$$\text{Specificity} = \frac{\text{True Negatives}}{\text{True Negatives} + \text{False Positives}}$$

Uncover the reliability of Genetic Testing through Sensitivity and Specificity calculations, distinguishing true positives, false negatives, true negatives, and false positives.

This section encapsulates Genetic Pediatric Diseases in Pediatric Pathology, presenting a quick and memorable overview enriched with diverse mathematical formulations and potential molecular/chemical equations.

14.4 Pediatric Infections

Embark on a swift exploration of Pediatric Infections in Pediatric Pathology, employing a succinct and memorable approach, incorporating various mathematical formulas and equations.

Immunization Coverage:

$$\text{Vaccination Coverage} = \frac{\text{Number of Vaccinated Individuals}}{\text{Total Population}} \times 100\%$$

Understand the significance of Immunization Coverage, a crucial metric calculated as the ratio of vaccinated individuals to the total population, expressed as a percentage.

Infection Transmission Rate:

$$\text{Transmission Rate} = \frac{\text{Number of New Cases}}{\text{Population at Risk}} \times 1000$$

Grasp the dynamics of infection spread with the Infection Transmission Rate, indicating the rate of new cases per thousand individuals in the population at risk.

Pediatric Antibiotic Dosage Calculation:

$$\text{Dosage} = \frac{\text{Child's Weight (kg)} \times \text{Desired Dose (mg/kg)}}{\text{Drug Concentration (mg/ml)}}$$

Navigate the realm of pediatric antibiotic administration with precision using the dosage calculation formula, incorporating the child's weight, desired dose, and drug concentration.

This section encapsulates Pediatric Infections in Pediatric Pathology, presenting a quick and memorable overview enriched with diverse mathematical formulations and potential molecular/chemical equations.

14.5   Tumors in Pediatrics

Embark on a rapid exploration of Pediatric Tumors in Pediatric Pathology, presenting a succinct and memorable overview incorporating diverse mathematical formulas and equations. Avoiding the use of dmath or align for plain texts, the focus is on delivering maximum content impact.

Tumor Incidence Rate:

$$\text{Incidence Rate} = \frac{\text{Number of New Cases}}{\text{Population at Risk}} \times 100,000$$

Understand the prevalence of Pediatric Tumors using the Incidence Rate, showcasing the rate of new cases per 100,000 individuals in the population at risk.

Survival Rate Calculation:

$$\text{Survival Rate} = \frac{\text{Number of Survivors}}{\text{Number of Cases}} \times 100\%$$

Navigate the landscape of Pediatric Tumor outcomes with the Survival Rate, a critical metric computed as the ratio of survivors to the total number of cases, expressed as a percentage.

Chemotherapy Dosage Calculation:

$$\text{Dosage} = \frac{\text{Patient's Body Surface Area (m}^2) \times \text{Desired Dose (mg/m}^2)}{\text{Drug Concentration (mg/ml)}}$$

Delve into the intricacies of chemotherapy dosage for pediatric tumors using the Dosage Calculation formula, incorporating the patient's body surface area, desired dose, and drug concentration.

This section encapsulates Pediatric Tumors in Pediatric Pathology, offering a quick and memorable overview enriched with various mathematical formulations and potential molecular/chemical equations.

14.6 Pediatric Laboratory Techniques

Embark on a swift exploration of Pediatric Laboratory Techniques in Pediatric Pathology, presenting a rapid and memorable overview incorporating diverse mathematical formulas and equations. Avoiding the use of dmath or align for plain texts, the focus is on delivering maximum content impact.

Laboratory Test Sensitivity and Specificity:

$$\text{Sensitivity} = \frac{\text{True Positives}}{\text{True Positives} + \text{False Negatives}} \times 100\%$$

$$\text{Specificity} = \frac{\text{True Negatives}}{\text{True Negatives} + \text{False Positives}} \times 100\%$$

Understand the diagnostic accuracy of laboratory tests using Sensitivity and Specificity, vital metrics calculated from true positive/negative and false positive/negative results.

Pediatric Blood Volume Calculation:

$$\text{Blood Volume} = \text{Weight (kg)} \times \text{Blood Volume Coefficient}$$

Navigate the intricacies of pediatric blood volume estimation using a simple formula based on the child's weight and a blood volume coefficient.

Molecular Diagnostic Techniques:

$$\text{PCR Amplification Efficiency} = (1 + \text{PCR Efficiency})^{(\text{Number of Cycles})}$$

Explore the efficiency of Polymerase Chain Reaction (PCR) amplification, a cornerstone in molecular diagnostics, using the PCR Amplification Efficiency formula.

This section encapsulates Pediatric Laboratory Techniques in Pediatric Pathology, offering a quick and memorable overview enriched with various mathematical formulations and potential molecular/chemical equations.

14.7 Pediatric Pathology Case Studies

Embark on a rapid journey through Pediatric Pathology Case Studies, employing diverse mathematical formulas and equations while refraining from using dmath or align for plain texts. This concise exploration aims to maximize content impact, potentially incorporating molecular or chemical equations.

Probability in Pediatric Disease:

$$P(A|B) = \frac{P(A \cap B)}{P(B)}$$

Utilize conditional probability to assess the likelihood of a pediatric disease (A) given certain conditions (B), employing the formula for conditional probability.

Genetic Risk Assessment:

$$\text{Risk} = \text{Baseline Risk} \times \text{Relative Risk}$$

Quantify the risk of pediatric diseases associated with genetics by employing the formula for risk assessment, incorporating baseline risk and relative risk.

Clinical Decision Support Systems (CDSS):

$$\text{Sensitivity} = \frac{\text{True Positives}}{\text{True Positives} + \text{False Negatives}}$$

Evaluate the performance of CDSS in pediatric pathology using sensitivity, a key metric calculated from true positive/negative and false positive/negative results.

This section encapsulates Pediatric Pathology Case Studies, providing a rapid and memorable overview enhanced with various mathematical formulas and equations, potentially incorporating molecular or chemical equations.

Chapter 15

Gynecological Pathology

15.1 Benign Gynecological Conditions

Embark on a rapid exploration of Benign Gynecological Conditions, employing various mathematical formulas and equations without dmath or align for plain texts. Maximize content impact, potentially incorporating molecular or chemical equations.

Fibroids Growth Rate:

$$\text{Volume} = \frac{4}{3}\pi r^3$$

Assess the growth rate of uterine fibroids using the formula for the volume of a sphere, where r represents the fibroid's radius.

Endometriosis Severity Score:

$$\text{ESS} = \sum (\text{Lesion Size} \times \text{Lesion Depth})$$

Quantify the severity of endometriosis with an Endometriosis Severity Score, computed by summing the product of lesion size and lesion depth.

Ovulation Prediction:

$$\text{Basal Body Temperature (BBT)} + \text{Luteinizing Hormone (LH)} Surge$$

Predict ovulation by monitoring basal body temperature (BBT) and detecting a surge in luteinizing hormone (LH).

This section provides a rapid, memorable overview of Benign Gynecological Conditions, incorporating various mathematical formulas and equations, potentially featuring molecular or chemical equations.

15.2 Gynecological Cancers

Embark on a swift exploration of Gynecological Cancers, leveraging a multitude of mathematical formulas and equations without dmath or align for plain texts. Feel free to integrate molecular or chemical equations for maximum content impact.

Risk Assessment for Ovarian Cancer:

$$\text{Risk} = \frac{\text{Number of Risk Factors}}{\text{Total Number of Factors Considered}} \times 100$$

Evaluate the risk of ovarian cancer by computing the ratio of risk factors to the total factors considered, expressed as a percentage.

HPV Transmission Probability:

$$\text{Transmission Probability} = 1 - (1 - \text{Transmission Rate})^{\text{Number of Contacts}}$$

Estimate the probability of Human Papillomavirus (HPV) transmission based on the transmission rate and the number of contacts.

Cervical Cancer Survival Rate:

$$\text{Survival Rate} = \frac{\text{Number of Survivors}}{\text{Total Number of Cases}} \times 100$$

Calculate the survival rate for cervical cancer by determining the ratio of survivors to the total number of cases, expressed as a percentage.

This section offers a rapid, memorable exploration of Gynecological Cancers, utilizing diverse mathematical formulas and equations, potentially incorporating molecular or chemical equations.

15.3 Reproductive System Infections

Delve into the realm of Reproductive System Infections, navigating through a concise and memorable exploration using an array of mathematical formulas and equations. Avoid dmath or align for plain texts, and feel free to incorporate molecular or chemical equations for an enriched presentation.

Incidence Rate of Vaginal Infections:

$$\text{Incidence Rate} = \frac{\text{Number of New Cases}}{\text{Population at Risk}} \times 1000$$

Calculate the incidence rate of vaginal infections by dividing the number of new cases by the population at risk, multiplied by 1000.

Treatment Efficacy for Endometritis:

$$\text{Efficacy} = \frac{\text{Number of Successful Treatments}}{\text{Total Number of Treatments}} \times 100$$

Assess the efficacy of endometritis treatment by determining the ratio of successful treatments to the total number of treatments, expressed as a percentage.

Antibiotic Dosage Calculation:

$$\text{Dosage} = \frac{\text{Patient's Weight} \times \text{Desired Dosage}}{\text{Concentration of Antibiotic}}$$

Compute the antibiotic dosage required based on the patient's weight, desired dosage, and the concentration of the antibiotic.

Embark on a swift journey through Reproductive System Infections, utilizing an array of mathematical formulas and equations, with potential integration of molecular or chemical equations for maximum impact.

15.4 Endometrial Pathology

Embark on a rapid exploration of Endometrial Pathology, employing a variety of mathematical formulas and equations, excluding dmath or align for plain texts. Consider incorporating molecular or chemical equations for added depth.

Endometrial Hyperplasia Risk Assessment:

$$\text{Relative Risk} = \frac{\text{Incidence in Exposed Group}}{\text{Incidence in Unexposed Group}}$$

Evaluate the relative risk of endometrial hyperplasia by comparing the incidence in an exposed group to that in an unexposed group.

Hormonal Therapy Success Rate:

$$\text{Success Rate} = \frac{\text{Number of Successful Cases}}{\text{Total Number of Cases}} \times 100$$

Determine the success rate of hormonal therapy for endometrial pathology by calculating the ratio of successful cases to the total number of cases, expressed as a percentage.

Estrogen Receptor (ER) Expression:

$$\text{ER Positivity Rate} = \frac{\text{Number of ER-Positive Cases}}{\text{Total Number of Cases}} \times 100$$

Explore the estrogen receptor (ER) positivity rate by examining the ratio of ER-positive cases to the total number of cases, presented as a percentage.

Embark on a swift journey through Endometrial Pathology, utilizing diverse mathematical expressions, and consider the inclusion of molecular or chemical equations for a comprehensive presentation.

15.5 Ovarian Pathology

Embark on a rapid exploration of Ovarian Pathology, utilizing a spectrum of mathematical formulas and equations, while avoiding dmath or align for plain texts. Molecular or chemical equations can be integrated if needed.

Ovarian Cancer Risk Calculation:

$$\text{Odds Ratio} = \frac{\text{Odds of Ovarian Cancer in Exposed Group}}{\text{Odds of Ovarian Cancer in Unexposed Group}}$$

Evaluate the odds ratio to assess the risk of ovarian cancer, comparing the odds in an exposed group to those in an unexposed group.

Ovarian Tumor Growth Rate:

$$\text{Tumor Growth Rate} = \frac{\text{Change in Tumor Size}}{\text{Time Interval}}$$

Calculate the ovarian tumor growth rate by dividing the change in tumor size by the time interval.

CA-125 Biomarker Sensitivity:

$$\text{Sensitivity} = \frac{\text{True Positive}}{\text{True Positive} + \text{False Negative}} \times 100$$

Assess the sensitivity of the CA-125 biomarker for ovarian pathology by determining the ratio of true positive cases to the sum of true positive and false negative cases, expressed as a percentage.

Embark on a swift journey through Ovarian Pathology, employing diverse mathematical expressions, and consider the inclusion of molecular or chemical equations for a comprehensive presentation.

15.6 Gynecological Pathology Case Studies

Immerse yourself in Gynecological Pathology through intriguing case studies, unraveling complexities with the aid of various mathematical formulas and equations. Employ dmath for specialized equations and incorporate molecular or chemical equations when necessary.

HPV Transmission Probability:

$$P(\text{Transmission}) = 1 - (1 - p)^n$$

Calculate the probability of human papillomavirus (HPV) transmission using the formula, where p is the probability of a single sexual encounter leading to transmission, and n is the number of sexual encounters.

Endometrial Biopsy Sensitivity:

$$\text{Sensitivity} = \frac{\text{True Positive}}{\text{True Positive} + \text{False Negative}} \times 100$$

Assess the sensitivity of endometrial biopsy in diagnosing pathologies by determining the ratio of true positive cases to the sum of true positive and false negative cases, expressed as a percentage.

Estrogen Receptor (ER) Status Ratio:

$$\text{ER Status Ratio} = \frac{\text{Number of ER-Positive Cases}}{\text{Number of ER-Negative Cases}}$$

Evaluate the estrogen receptor (ER) status ratio to understand the prevalence of ER-positive and ER-negative cases in gynecological pathologies.

Embark on a captivating journey through Gynecological Pathology case studies, employing diverse mathematical expressions, and considering the inclusion of molecular or chemical equations for a comprehensive presentation.

Chapter 16

Urological Pathology

16.1 Benign Prostatic Diseases

Delve into the realm of Urological Pathology, specifically exploring the intricacies of Benign Prostatic Diseases. Leverage a variety of mathematical formulas and equations, utilizing dmath for specialized expressions, and consider incorporating molecular or chemical equations when relevant.

Prostate Volume Calculation:

$$V = \frac{1}{6}\pi h \left(3r^2 + h^2\right)$$

Compute the volume of the prostate using the formula, where V is the volume, π is a mathematical constant, h is the height, and r is the radius.

Prostate-Specific Antigen (PSA) Density:

$$\text{PSA Density} = \frac{\text{PSA Level}}{\text{Prostate Volume}}$$

Evaluate the PSA density by dividing the PSA level by the prostate volume, providing insights into the concentration of PSA in relation to prostate size.

Bladder Capacity Estimation:

$$\text{Bladder Capacity} = \frac{\text{Voided Volume} + \text{Post-Void Residual}}{2}$$

Estimate the bladder capacity by averaging the voided volume and post-void residual, contributing to a comprehensive understanding of bladder health.

Immerse yourself in the world of Benign Prostatic Diseases within Urological Pathology, employing diverse mathematical expressions and potential molecular or chemical equations for a thorough presentation.

16.2 Prostate Cancer

Embark on the exploration of Prostate Cancer within the domain of Urological Pathology, unraveling complexities in a concise and memorable manner. Employ a variety of mathematical formulas and equations, utilizing dmath for specialized expressions. Consider incorporating molecular or chemical equations when relevant.

Gleason Score Calculation:

$$\text{Gleason Score} = \text{Primary Grade} + \text{Secondary Grade}$$

Determine the Gleason Score by summing up the primary and secondary grades, providing a comprehensive assessment of prostate cancer aggressiveness.

Prostate-Specific Antigen (PSA) Velocity:

$$\text{PSA Velocity} = \frac{\Delta \text{PSA}}{\Delta \text{Time}}$$

Calculate the PSA velocity by dividing the change in PSA (ΔPSA) by the change in time (ΔTime), aiding in the evaluation of the rate of PSA level changes.

TNM Staging System:

$$\text{Tumor Size} \times \text{Node Involvement} \times \text{Metastasis Presence}$$

Utilize the TNM staging system, multiplying factors related to tumor size, node involvement, and metastasis presence for a comprehensive prostate cancer stage assessment.

Immerse yourself in the intricacies of Prostate Cancer in Urological Pathology, employing diverse mathematical expressions and potential molecular or chemical equations for a robust presentation.

16.3 Renal and Bladder Pathology

Embark on the exploration of Renal and Bladder Pathology within the domain of Urological Pathology, unraveling complexities in a concise and memorable manner. Employ a variety of mathematical formulas and equations, utilizing dmath for specialized expressions. Consider incorporating molecular or chemical equations when relevant.

Glomerular Filtration Rate (GFR) Calculation:

$$\text{GFR} = \frac{k \times \text{Creatinine}}{\text{Age}}$$

Determine the Glomerular Filtration Rate (GFR) by multiplying a constant (k) with the creatinine level and dividing by the age, providing insights into renal function.

Bladder Capacity Calculation:

$$\text{Bladder Capacity} = \frac{\text{Voided Volume} + \text{Residual Volume}}{\text{Number of Voids}}$$

Calculate the Bladder Capacity by summing the voided volume and residual volume, divided by the number of voids, offering a measure of bladder function.

Nephron-Sparing Surgery Criteria:

$$\text{Tumor Size} + \text{Solitary Kidney} + \text{Bilateral Tumors}$$

Utilize the Nephron-Sparing Surgery criteria, considering factors such as tumor size, solitary kidney status, and presence of bilateral tumors for decision-making in renal surgeries.

Immerse yourself in the intricacies of Renal and Bladder Pathology in Urological Pathology, employing diverse mathematical expressions and potential molecular or chemical equations for a robust presentation.

16.4   Testicular Pathology

Embark on the exploration of Testicular Pathology within the domain of Urological Pathology, elucidating complexities in a succinct and memorable manner. Employ a variety of mathematical formulas and equations, utilizing dmath for specialized expressions. Consider incorporating molecular or chemical equations when relevant.

Testicular Volume Calculation:

$$\text{Volume} = \frac{4}{3}\pi r^3$$

Compute the testicular volume using the formula for the volume of a sphere, where r is the radius.

Sperm Count Calculation:

$$\text{Sperm Count} = \frac{\text{Total Sperm Count}}{\text{Volume of Ejaculate}}$$

Determine the sperm count by dividing the total sperm count by the volume of ejaculate, providing insights into male fertility.

Testicular Tumor Marker:

$$\text{AFP (Alpha-Fetoprotein)}$$

Consider the Alpha-Fetoprotein (AFP) as a tumor marker for testicular tumors, aiding in diagnosis and monitoring.

Immerse yourself in the intricacies of Testicular Pathology in Urological Pathology, employing diverse mathematical expressions and potential molecular or chemical equations for a comprehensive presentation.

16.5 Urological Infections

Delve into the realm of Urological Infections within Urological Pathology, simplifying complexities with mathematical formulas and equations, utilizing dmath for specialized expressions. Integrate molecular or chemical equations when pertinent.

Calculation of Urinary Tract Infection (UTI) Risk:

$$\text{UTI Risk} = \frac{\text{Number of Pathogens} \times \text{Virulence}}{\text{Host Resistance}}$$

Estimate the risk of Urinary Tract Infection (UTI) by considering the number of pathogens, their virulence, and the host's resistance.

Antibiotic Dosage Calculation:

$$\text{Dosage} = \frac{\text{Patient's Weight} \times \text{Desired Concentration}}{\text{Drug Concentration}}$$

Compute the appropriate antibiotic dosage based on the patient's weight, desired concentration, and drug concentration.

Chemical Equation for Antibacterial Action:

$$\text{Antibacterial Agent} + \text{Pathogen} \rightarrow \text{Inactive Compounds} + \text{Harmless Byproducts}$$

Illustrate the antibacterial action using a chemical equation, showcasing the transformation of antibacterial agents and pathogens into inactive compounds and harmless byproducts.

Immerse yourself in the intricacies of Urological Infections in Urological Pathology, leveraging mathematical expressions and potential molecular or chemical equations for a comprehensive understanding.

16.6 Urological Pathology Case Studies

Embark on a journey through Urological Pathology Case Studies, unraveling complexities with concise mathematical formulations and equations. Employ dmath for specialized expressions and seamlessly integrate molecular or chemical equations when needed.

Calculation of Renal Function:

$$\text{Glomerular Filtration Rate (GFR)} = \frac{k \times \text{Creatinine}}{\text{Serum Creatinine}}$$

Determine the Glomerular Filtration Rate (GFR) by applying the appropriate constant (k) to the ratio of creatinine and serum creatinine.

Risk Assessment for Bladder Cancer:

$$\text{Risk} = \frac{\text{Exposure Level} \times \text{Genetic Predisposition}}{\text{Detoxification Capacity}}$$

Evaluate the risk of bladder cancer by considering exposure levels, genetic predisposition, and the detoxification capacity of the patient.

Chemical Equation for Kidney Stones Formation:

$$\text{Calcium} + \text{Oxalate} \rightarrow \text{Calcium Oxalate}$$

Represent the formation of kidney stones through a chemical equation involving the reaction between calcium and oxalate, resulting in calcium oxalate.

Immerse yourself in Urological Pathology Case Studies, navigating through mathematical insights and potential molecular or chemical equations for an enriched understanding.

Chapter 17

Neuropathology

17.1 Neurodegenerative Diseases

Delve into the realm of Neurodegenerative Diseases, unraveling complexities through succinct mathematical formulations and equations. Employ dmath for specialized expressions and seamlessly integrate molecular or chemical equations when necessary.

Calculation of Alzheimer's Disease Risk:

$$\text{Risk} = \frac{\text{Genetic Factors} \times \text{Age}}{\text{Protective Factors}}$$

Estimate the risk of Alzheimer's disease by considering genetic factors, age, and protective factors that may mitigate the risk.

Neuronal Loss in Parkinson's Disease:

$$\text{Neuronal Loss} = \text{Initial Neuronal Count} - (\text{Rate of Neuronal Death} \times \text{Time})$$

Quantify neuronal loss in Parkinson's disease by subtracting the product of the rate of neuronal death and time from the initial neuronal count.

Chemical Basis of Prion Diseases:

$$\text{Normal Prion Protein } (\text{PrP}^{C}) \rightleftharpoons \text{Abnormal Prion Protein } (\text{PrP}^{Sc})$$

Describe the chemical equilibrium between normal (PrP^{C}) and abnormal (PrP^{Sc}) prion proteins, central to the pathogenesis of prion diseases.

Embark on a journey through Neurodegenerative Diseases, exploring mathematical insights and potential molecular or chemical equations for a comprehensive understanding.

17.2 Central Nervous System Tumors

Embark on the exploration of Central Nervous System (CNS) Tumors, unraveling complexities through concise mathematical formulations and equations. Leverage dmath for specialized expressions and seamlessly integrate molecular or chemical equations when necessary.

Growth Rate of CNS Tumors:

$$\text{Volume} = \frac{4}{3}\pi r^3$$

$$\text{Doubling Time} = \frac{\ln(2)}{\text{Growth Rate}}$$

Understand the growth of CNS tumors by calculating their volume using the sphere formula. Determine the doubling time, a critical parameter in assessing tumor aggressiveness.

Tumor Suppressor Gene Action:

$$\text{Tumor Suppressor Gene} \xrightarrow{\text{Mutation}} \text{Loss of Function}$$

Explore the impact of mutations on tumor suppressor genes, leading to the loss of their normal function, a key mechanism in the development of CNS tumors.

Chemotherapy Drug Interaction:

$$\text{Drug A} + \text{Drug B} \xrightarrow{\text{Synergy}} \text{Enhanced Efficacy}$$

Examine the synergy between chemotherapy drugs A and B, highlighting how their combination can result in enhanced efficacy against CNS tumors.

Embark on a mathematical journey through CNS Tumors, deciphering growth dynamics, genetic influences, and potential drug interactions.

17.3 Vascular Disorders of the Brain

Delve into the intricacies of Vascular Disorders of the Brain using succinct mathematical formulations and equations, leveraging dmath for clarity. Integrate molecular or chemical equations seamlessly when needed.

Cerebral Blood Flow (CBF) Calculation:

$$CBF = \frac{\Delta Q}{\Delta P}$$

Understand the dynamics of Cerebral Blood Flow (CBF) by calculating it as the ratio of the change in blood quantity (ΔQ) to the change in pressure (ΔP).

Ischemic Stroke Risk Prediction:

$$\text{Risk} = \frac{\text{Blood Viscosity} \times \text{Plaque Formation}}{\text{Vessel Diameter}}$$

Evaluate the risk of ischemic stroke by considering factors such as blood viscosity, plaque formation, and vessel diameter, providing insights into preventive measures.

Hemorrhagic Stroke Severity Index:

$$\text{Severity Index} = \frac{\text{Volume of Bleeding}}{\text{Brain Volume}} \times 100$$

Assess the severity of hemorrhagic stroke using the Severity Index, calculated as the ratio of the volume of bleeding to the total brain volume, expressed as a percentage.

Embark on a mathematical exploration of Vascular Disorders of the Brain, unraveling the complexities of cerebral blood flow, stroke risk, and hemorrhagic stroke severity.

17.4 Infectious Diseases of the Nervous System

Dive into the realm of Infectious Diseases of the Nervous System, unraveling the complexities through concise mathematical expressions and equations, leveraging dmath for clarity. Integrate molecular or chemical equations seamlessly when needed.

Neuroinvasion Probability:

$$P(\text{Neuroinvasion}) = \frac{\text{Viral Load in CNS}}{\text{Immune Response}}$$

Explore the likelihood of neuroinvasion by calculating the probability as the ratio of the viral load in the central nervous system (CNS) to the strength of the immune response.

Inflammatory Response Dynamics:

$$\frac{d(\text{Inflammation})}{dt} = \text{Infection Rate} - \text{Clearance Rate}$$

Understand the dynamics of the inflammatory response by considering the rate of infection and the rate of clearance over time.

Meningitis Risk Score:

$$\text{Risk Score} = \frac{\text{Pathogen Virulence} \times \text{Host Susceptibility}}{\text{Immune Response}}$$

Assess the risk of meningitis by combining factors such as pathogen virulence, host susceptibility, and the strength of the immune response.

Embark on a mathematical exploration of Infectious Diseases of the Nervous System, shedding light on neuroinvasion, inflammatory response dynamics, and meningitis risk.

17.5   Neuromuscular Pathology

Embark on the journey through Neuromuscular Pathology, unraveling its intricacies through succinct mathematical expressions and equations, employing dmath for clarity. Seamless integration of molecular or chemical equations enriches the depth of understanding.

Muscle Contraction Dynamics:

$$Tension(t) = \int_0^t \left(\frac{\partial Ca^{2+}}{\partial t} \times \text{Contractile Element Sensitivity} \right) dt$$

Explore the dynamics of muscle contraction by calculating tension as the integral of the rate of change of calcium ion concentration with respect to time, multiplied by contractile element sensitivity.

Motor Unit Firing Rate:

$$FiringRate = \frac{\text{Motor Neuron Excitability}}{\text{Synaptic Input Resistance}}$$

Understand motor unit firing rates by considering the ratio of motor neuron excitability to synaptic input resistance.

Neuromuscular Transmission Efficiency:

$$Efficiency = \frac{\text{Number of Released Quanta}}{\text{Number of Motor Endplate Receptors}}$$

Assess neuromuscular transmission efficiency by calculating the ratio of the number of released quanta to the number of motor endplate receptors.

Embark on a mathematical exploration of Neuromuscular Pathology, delving into muscle contraction dynamics, motor unit firing rates, and neuromuscular transmission efficiency.

17.6   Neuropathology Case Studies

Embark on a journey through Neuropathology Case Studies, deciphering intricate details with the aid of mathematical expressions and equations, employing dmath for clarity. Seamlessly integrate molecular or chemical equations when necessary.

Neurological Assessment Score:

$$\text{Neuro Score} = \frac{\text{Motor Function} + \text{Sensory Response} + \text{Cognitive Ability}}{\text{Age Factor}}$$

Evaluate the neurological status using a comprehensive Neuro Score that considers motor function, sensory response, and cognitive ability, normalized by an age factor.

Disease Progression Rate:

$$\frac{d(\text{Disease Severity})}{dt} = \text{Inflammatory Response} - \text{Treatment Efficacy}$$

Track the progression of neuropathological diseases by assessing the rate of change in disease severity, influenced by the balance between inflammatory response and treatment efficacy.

Neuropathological Scoring System:

$$\text{Neuro Score} = \frac{\text{Extent of Lesion} \times \text{Degree of Necrosis}}{\text{Regeneration Potential}}$$

Develop a scoring system for neuropathological conditions, factoring in the extent of lesions, degree of necrosis, and the regeneration potential of neural tissues.

Delve into Neuropathology Case Studies armed with mathematical tools, unraveling the complexities of neurological assessment, disease progression, and a comprehensive scoring system.

Chapter 18

Musculoskeletal Pathology

18.1 Bone Diseases

Uncover the intricacies of Bone Diseases in Musculoskeletal Pathology through concise mathematical expressions and equations, leveraging the power of dmath for clarity. Molecular or chemical equations seamlessly integrate to elucidate complex concepts.

Bone Mineral Density (BMD):

$$\text{BMD} = \frac{\text{Mass of Minerals in Bone}}{\text{Bone Volume}}$$

Evaluate Bone Mineral Density (BMD) by discerning the ratio of the mass of minerals in bone to the bone volume, providing valuable insights into bone health.

Fracture Risk Assessment:

$$\text{Fracture Risk} = \text{BMD} - \frac{\text{Age Factor} \times \text{Body Mass Index (BMI)}}{\text{Previous Fracture History}}$$

Assess fracture risk comprehensively using a formula that incorporates BMD, age factor, BMI, and previous fracture history.

Osteoclast Activity:

$$\text{Osteoclast Activity} = \frac{\text{Number of Active Osteoclasts}}{\text{Bone Surface Area}}$$

Quantify osteoclast activity by determining the ratio of active osteoclasts to the bone surface area, a key metric in understanding bone remodeling.

Embark on the exploration of Bone Diseases armed with mathematical tools, unraveling the nuances of Bone Mineral Density, Fracture Risk, and Osteoclast Activity.

18.2   Joint Disorders

Delve into the realm of Joint Disorders in Musculoskeletal Pathology, unraveling the complexities through concise mathematical expressions and equations. Leverage the clarity of dmath without cumbersome alignments for plain texts. Molecular or chemical equations seamlessly integrate to enhance the understanding of intricate concepts.

Articular Cartilage Health:

$$\text{Articular Cartilage Health} = \frac{\text{GAG Content}}{\text{Collagen Content}}$$

Evaluate the health of articular cartilage by examining the ratio of Glycosaminoglycan (GAG) content to Collagen content, providing insights into the composition of cartilage.

Joint Range of Motion (ROM):

$$\text{Joint ROM} = \frac{\text{Final Joint Position} - \text{Initial Joint Position}}{\text{Time}}$$

Assess Joint Range of Motion by calculating the change in joint position over time, a crucial metric in understanding joint flexibility.

Synovial Fluid Viscosity:

$$\text{Synovial Fluid Viscosity} = \frac{\text{Shear Stress}}{\text{Shear Rate}}$$

Understand the viscosity of synovial fluid by determining the ratio of shear stress to shear rate, impacting joint lubrication and function.

Embark on a mathematical journey through Joint Disorders, exploring Articular Cartilage Health, Joint Range of Motion, and Synovial Fluid Viscosity.

18.3   Soft Tissue Pathology

Dive into the intricacies of Soft Tissue Pathology within Musculoskeletal Pathology, deciphering complex concepts through succinct mathematical expressions and equations. Opt for the clarity of dmath without cumbersome alignments for plain texts. Molecular or chemical equations seamlessly integrate to augment the understanding of nuanced ideas.

Tumor Growth Rate:

$$\text{Tumor Growth Rate} = \frac{\text{Change in Tumor Size}}{\text{Time}}$$

Unravel the dynamics of tumor development by calculating the Tumor Growth Rate, providing crucial insights into the progression of soft tissue tumors.

Stress-Strain Relationship:

$$\sigma = \frac{F}{A} \quad \varepsilon = \frac{\Delta L}{L_0}$$

Explore the Stress-Strain Relationship to comprehend how soft tissues respond to external forces, utilizing stress (σ) and strain (ε) equations.

Soft Tissue Healing:

$$\text{Healing Rate} = \frac{\text{Change in Tissue Integrity}}{\text{Time}}$$

Evaluate the rate of soft tissue healing by analyzing the change in tissue integrity over time, a crucial parameter in understanding recovery.

Embark on a mathematical journey through Soft Tissue Pathology, exploring Tumor Growth Rate, the Stress-Strain Relationship, and Soft Tissue Healing.

18.4 Musculoskeletal Infections

Delve into the realm of Musculoskeletal Infections, decoding intricate concepts with concise mathematical expressions and equations. Utilize the power of dmath without the complexity of alignments for plain texts. Molecular or chemical equations seamlessly integrate to enhance the understanding of infectious processes.

Infection Severity Index:

$$\text{Infection Severity Index} = \frac{\text{Extent of Infection}}{\text{Time}}$$

Quantify the severity of musculoskeletal infections by calculating the Infection Severity Index, highlighting the relationship between the extent of infection and time.

Antibiotic Efficacy:

$$\text{Efficacy} = 1 - e^{-k \cdot t}$$

Understand the efficacy of antibiotics in treating musculoskeletal infections with the Antibiotic Efficacy formula, where k is the rate constant and t is time.

Host Immune Response:

$$\text{Immune Response} = \frac{\text{Activated Immune Cells}}{\text{Total Immune Cells}}$$

Explore the dynamics of the host immune response in musculoskeletal infections, assessing the ratio of activated immune cells to the total immune cell population.

Embark on a mathematical exploration of Musculoskeletal Infections, covering the Infection Severity Index, Antibiotic Efficacy, and Host Immune Response.

18.5　Tumors of the Musculoskeletal System

Unveil the intricacies of Musculoskeletal Tumors through a concise and memorable lens, employing mathematical formulas and equations without the complexities of alignments.

Tumor Growth Rate:

$$\text{Growth Rate} = \frac{\Delta \text{Tumor Size}}{\Delta \text{Time}}$$

Decipher the pace of tumor development with the Tumor Growth Rate formula, where ΔTumor Size represents the change in tumor size over time.

Probability of Metastasis:

$$\text{Probability} = \frac{\text{Number of Metastatic Sites}}{\text{Total Number of Sites}} \times 100$$

Quantify the likelihood of metastasis using the Probability of Metastasis formula, expressing the ratio of metastatic sites to the total number of sites as a percentage.

Genetic Susceptibility:

$$\text{Risk} = \text{Baseline Risk} \times \text{Genetic Factor}$$

Explore the influence of genetic factors on tumor development with the Genetic Susceptibility formula, indicating the increased risk associated with specific genetic factors.

Delve into the realm of Musculoskeletal Tumors, utilizing mathematical expressions for Tumor Growth Rate, Probability of Metastasis, and Genetic Susceptibility.

18.6　Musculoskeletal Pathology Case Studies

Embark on a journey through Musculoskeletal Pathology Case Studies, unraveling complexities with the aid of mathematical formulations and chemical equations.

Clinical Assessment Score:

$$\text{Clinical Score} = \sum_{i=1}^{n} \left(\frac{\text{Parameter}_i}{\text{Maximum Value}_i} \right) \times 100$$

Evaluate the severity of musculoskeletal conditions using the Clinical Assessment Score, amalgamating various parameters and their respective maximum values.

Response to Treatment Index:

$$\text{Response Index} = \frac{\text{Post-treatment Measurement} - \text{Pre-treatment Measurement}}{\text{Pre-treatment Measurement}} \times 100$$

Quantify the efficacy of treatments through the Response to Treatment Index, expressing the percentage change in measurements before and after treatment.

Chemical Reaction of Therapeutic Agent:

$$\text{Drug} + \text{Target} \xleftrightarrow{k_1} k_{-1}\text{Drug-Target Complex} \xrightarrow{k_2} \text{Product}$$

Illuminate the pharmacological landscape with the chemical reaction governing the interaction between a therapeutic drug and its target, unveiling the formation of a drug-target complex and subsequent product generation.

Embark on Musculoskeletal Pathology Case Studies, employing mathematical tools for Clinical Assessment, Treatment Response, and delving into chemical reactions of therapeutic agents.

Chapter 19

Otolaryngologic Pathology

19.1   Ear Pathology

Embark on the fascinating journey of Ear Pathology, exploring its intricacies through a lens of mathematical formulas and equations, avoiding complex alignments and utilizing molecular or chemical equations when necessary.

Sound Intensity:

$$I = \frac{P^2}{A}$$

Delve into the realm of sound with the Sound Intensity formula, where I represents intensity, P is the sound pressure, and A denotes the area.

Frequency-Wavelength Relationship:

$$v = f\lambda$$

Uncover the relationship between frequency (f) and wavelength (λ) with the Frequency-Wavelength formula, where v is the speed of sound.

Otosclerosis Risk Assessment:

$$\text{Risk} = \frac{\text{Age} \times \text{Family History}}{\text{Calcium Metabolism}}$$

Assess the risk of otosclerosis using the Otosclerosis Risk Assessment formula, considering factors like age, family history, and calcium metabolism.

Chemical Reaction in Ear Infections:

$$\text{Reactants} \xrightarrow{\text{Conditions}} \text{Products}$$

For a comprehensive understanding, visualize chemical reactions involved in ear infections, showcasing reactants transforming into products under specific conditions.

Embark on the mathematical and chemical odyssey of Ear Pathology, assimilating diverse content for a holistic perspective.

19.2   Nose and Sinus Pathology

Embark on the exploration of Nose and Sinus Pathology, unraveling its complexities through concise mathematical formulations and equations, avoiding complex alignments, and incorporating molecular or chemical equations as needed.

Nasal Airflow Resistance:

$$R = \frac{\Delta P}{\dot{V}}$$

Dive into the dynamics of nasal airflow with the Nasal Airflow Resistance formula, where R signifies resistance, ΔP is the pressure difference, and $\dot{V}$ represents airflow.

Sinusitis Severity Index (SSI):

$$\text{SSI} = \text{Purulence} + \text{Ostial Obstruction} + \text{CT Findings}$$

Evaluate the severity of sinusitis using the Sinusitis Severity Index (SSI), a composite score incorporating factors like purulence, ostial obstruction, and CT findings.

Chemical Mediators in Allergic Rhinitis:

$$\text{Allergen} + \text{Mast Cells} \xrightarrow{\text{Activation}} \text{Chemical Mediators}$$

Visualize the cascade of allergic reactions in rhinitis, as allergens interact with mast cells, leading to the release of chemical mediators.

Uncover the intricacies of Nose and Sinus Pathology through a blend of mathematical precision and chemical insights, providing a comprehensive overview of the subject.

19.3   Throat and Larynx Pathology

Embark on the exploration of Throat and Larynx Pathology, unraveling its intricacies through concise mathematical formulations and equations, avoiding complex alignments, and incorporating molecular or chemical equations as needed.

Vocal Fold Vibration Frequency:

$$f = \frac{T}{2}$$

Delve into the dynamics of vocal fold vibration, where f represents frequency and T signifies the period.

Laryngeal Cancer Staging (TNM):

$$\text{TNM Stage} = \text{Tumor Size} + \text{Node Involvement} + \text{Metastasis Presence}$$

Understand the staging of laryngeal cancer using the TNM system, combining factors such as tumor size, node involvement, and metastasis presence.

Laryngopharyngeal Reflux (LPR) Index:

$$\text{LPR Index} = \frac{\text{Number of Reflux Episodes}}{\text{Duration of Monitoring}}$$

Explore the Laryngopharyngeal Reflux (LPR) Index, a metric derived from the ratio of reflux episodes to the duration of monitoring.

Uncover the complexities of Throat and Larynx Pathology through a blend of mathematical precision and formulaic insights, providing a comprehensive overview of the subject.

19.4 Head and Neck Tumors

Embark on the journey through Head and Neck Tumors, navigating their intricacies with succinct mathematical formulations and equations. Steer clear of complex alignments, and introduce molecular or chemical equations where appropriate for a comprehensive exploration.

Tumor Growth Model:

$$V(t) = V_0 e^{rt}$$

Embark on the understanding of tumor growth dynamics with the Tumor Growth Model, where $V(t)$ denotes the tumor volume at time t, V_0 is the initial volume, r is the growth rate.

TNM Staging System:

$$\text{Stage} = \text{T} + \text{N} + \text{M}$$

Unravel the staging of tumors with the TNM Staging System, a summation of factors like tumor size (T), lymph node involvement (N), and distant metastasis (M).

Chemotherapy Drug Interaction:

$$\text{Drug}_1 + \text{Drug}_2 \xrightarrow{\text{Interaction}} \text{Effect}$$

Delve into the interactions of chemotherapy drugs, where the combination of Drug_1 and Drug_2 leads to a specific therapeutic effect.

Embark on a mathematical journey through the realm of Head and Neck Tumors, unveiling their secrets through formulas and equations, providing a concise yet comprehensive overview.

19.5 Infections of the Otolaryngologic System

Embark on a concise exploration of Infections of the Otolaryngologic System, employing mathematical expressions and chemical equations for a rapid grasp.

Infection Severity Index:

$$\text{Severity} = \frac{\text{Symptom Score} \times \text{Pathogen Load}}{\text{Immune Response}}$$

Navigate the landscape of infection severity using the Infection Severity Index, combining Symptom Score, Pathogen Load, and Immune Response.

Antibiotic Effectiveness:

$$\text{Bacterial Load}_{\text{Post-Treatment}} = \text{Bacterial Load}_{\text{Pre-Treatment}} \times (1 - \text{Drug Efficacy})$$

Dive into antibiotic effectiveness calculations, where the post-treatment bacterial load relates to the pre-treatment load and drug efficacy.

Viral Replication Model:

$$V(t) = V_0 e^{rt}$$

Unlock the dynamics of viral replication with the Viral Replication Model, showcasing the viral load ($V(t)$), initial load (V_0), growth rate (r), and time (t).

Embark on a mathematical journey through the intricacies of Otolaryngologic System Infections, gaining insights with formulas and equations for a swift understanding.

19.6 Otolaryngologic Pathology Case Studies

Embark on a journey through Otolaryngologic Pathology Case Studies, unraveling complexities with mathematical expressions and chemical equations.

Disease Progression Model:

$$\text{Severity}_{\text{Time}} = \frac{\text{Symptom Load}}{\text{Time}}$$

Illuminate the Disease Progression Model, capturing the evolving severity ($\text{Severity}_{\text{Time}}$) concerning Symptom Load and Time.

Treatment Efficacy Index:

$$\text{Efficacy} = \frac{\text{Post-Treatment Improvement}}{\text{Pre-Treatment Condition}}$$

Delve into the Treatment Efficacy Index, quantifying efficacy based on Post-Treatment Improvement and Pre-Treatment Condition.

Genetic Susceptibility Equation:

$$\text{Risk} = \text{Baseline Risk} \times \left(1 + \frac{\text{Genetic Factor}}{100}\right)$$

Uncover the Genetic Susceptibility Equation, estimating risk considering the Baseline Risk and the influence of a Genetic Factor.

Molecular Interaction in Pathogenesis:

$$A + B \underset{k_{-1}}{\overset{k_1}{\rightleftharpoons}} C$$

Peer into the molecular realm with a chemical equation depicting the interaction ($A + B \underset{k_{-1}}{\overset{k_1}{\rightleftharpoons}} C$) influencing pathogenesis.

Embark on a mathematical and molecular exploration of Otolaryngologic Pathology Case Studies, enhancing comprehension with diverse formulas and equations.

Chapter 20

Cardiac Pathology

20.1 Ischemic Heart Disease

Embark on a journey through Ischemic Heart Disease, exploring complexities through mathematical formulas and chemical equations.

Cardiac Output Equation:

$$\text{Cardiac Output} = \text{Heart Rate} \times \text{Stroke Volume}$$

Uncover the Cardiac Output Equation, defining the cardiac output as the product of heart rate and stroke volume.

Myocardial Oxygen Demand:

$$\text{MVO}_2 = \text{Heart Rate} \times \text{Systolic Blood Pressure} \times \text{Myocardial Contractility}$$

Dive into the Myocardial Oxygen Demand formula (MVO_2), capturing the intricate relationship with heart rate, systolic blood pressure, and myocardial contractility.

Ischemic Injury Threshold:

$$\text{Ischemic Injury} = \frac{\text{Myocardial Oxygen Supply}}{\text{Myocardial Oxygen Demand}}$$

Illuminate the Ischemic Injury Threshold, exploring the delicate balance between myocardial oxygen supply and demand.

Chemical Reaction in Ischemia:

$$\text{Glucose} + \text{Oxygen} \xrightarrow[\text{Ischemia}]{\text{Anaerobic Conditions}} \text{Lactic Acid}$$

Peer into the molecular level with a chemical equation (Glucose + Oxygen $\xrightarrow[\text{Ischemia}]{\text{Anaerobic Conditions}}$ Lactic Acid) depicting reactions during ischemic conditions.

Embark on a mathematical and molecular exploration of Ischemic Heart Disease, enhancing understanding with diverse formulas and equations.

20.2 Valvular Heart Diseases

Embark on a journey through Valvular Heart Diseases, unraveling complexities through mathematical formulas and chemical equations.

Valve Area Calculation (for Stenosis):

$$\text{Valve Area} = \frac{\text{Flow Rate}}{\text{Velocity of Blood Through Valve}}$$

Delve into the Valve Area Calculation, a crucial formula determining the valve area based on flow rate and velocity of blood through the valve.

Regurgitant Fraction (for Regurgitation):

$$\text{Regurgitant Fraction} = \frac{\text{Regurgitant Volume}}{\text{Stroke Volume}}$$

Explore the Regurgitant Fraction, a mathematical representation of regurgitation, defined as the ratio of regurgitant volume to stroke volume.

Bernoulli's Equation:

$$\text{Pressure Drop} = 4 \times \left(\frac{\text{Velocity}}{2}\right)^2$$

Uncover Bernoulli's Equation, an essential formula describing the pressure drop across a stenotic valve, emphasizing the relationship with velocity.

Chemical Reaction in Valvular Dysfunction:

$$\text{Calcium Deposits} + \text{Inflammatory Mediators} \xrightarrow{\text{Valvular Dysfunction}} \text{Valve Degeneration}$$

Peer into the molecular level with a chemical equation

(Calcium Deposits + Inflammatory Mediators $\xrightarrow{\text{Valvular Dysfunction}}$ Valve Degeneration) depicting reactions leading to valvular dysfunction.

Embark on a mathematical and molecular exploration of Valvular Heart Diseases, enhancing understanding with diverse formulas and equations.

20.3 Cardiomyopathies

Embark on the exploration of Cardiomyopathies, unraveling complexities through mathematical formulas and chemical equations.

Ejection Fraction (EF):

$$EF = \frac{\text{End-Diastolic Volume (EDV) - End-Systolic Volume (ESV)}}{\text{End-Diastolic Volume (EDV)}} \times 100\%$$

Dive into the Ejection Fraction (EF), a vital indicator of cardiac performance, calculated as the percentage of blood pumped out of the heart with each contraction.

Hemodynamic Stress:

$$\text{Stress} = \frac{\text{Pressure}}{\text{Wall Thickness}}$$

Explore Hemodynamic Stress, a mathematical representation of the stress imposed on the heart wall, defined as the ratio of pressure to wall thickness.

Chemical Pathway in Cardiomyopathies:

$$\text{Genetic Factors} + \text{Environmental Triggers} \xrightarrow{\text{Cardiomyopathies}} \text{Myocardial Damage}$$

Peer into the molecular level with a chemical equation

$$(\text{Genetic Factors} + \text{Environmental Triggers} \xrightarrow{\text{Cardiomyopathies}} \text{Myocardial Damage})$$ depicting factors contributing to cardiomyopathies.

Embark on a mathematical and molecular journey through Cardiomyopathies, enhancing understanding with diverse formulas and equations.

20.4 Congenital Heart Diseases

Embark on the exploration of Congenital Heart Diseases, unraveling complexities through mathematical formulas and chemical equations.

Shunt Fraction (Qp/Qs):

$$Qp/Qs = \frac{\text{Pulmonary Blood Flow (Qp)}}{\text{Systemic Blood Flow (Qs)}}$$

Dive into the Shunt Fraction (Qp/Qs), a crucial parameter in congenital heart diseases, calculated as the ratio of pulmonary blood flow to systemic blood flow.

Cardiac Output (CO):

$$CO = \text{Heart Rate} \times \text{Stroke Volume}$$

Explore Cardiac Output (CO), a fundamental measure reflecting the volume of blood the heart pumps per minute, derived from heart rate and stroke volume.

Chemical Pathway in Congenital Heart Diseases:

$$\text{Genetic Factors} + \text{Environmental Influences} \xrightarrow{\text{Congenital Heart Diseases}} \text{Cardiac Anomalies}$$

Peer into the molecular level with a chemical equation

$$(\text{Genetic Factors} + \text{Environmental Influences} \xrightarrow{\text{Congenital Heart Diseases}} \text{Cardiac Anomalies})$$

illustrating the interplay leading to congenital heart diseases.

Embark on a mathematical and molecular journey through Congenital Heart Diseases, enhancing understanding with diverse formulas and equations.

20.5 Cardiac Infections

Embark on a rapid exploration of Cardiac Infections, unraveling complexities with mathematical formulas and chemical equations.

Infection Severity Index (ISI):

$$ISI = \frac{\text{Cardiac Inflammatory Markers (CIM)}}{\text{Cardiac Function Index (CFI)}}$$

Dive into the Infection Severity Index (ISI), a critical measure in cardiac infections, calculated as the ratio of cardiac inflammatory markers to cardiac function index.

Cardiac Infection Model:

$$\text{Pathogen} + \text{Host Factors} \xrightarrow{\text{Cardiac Infection}} \text{Inflammatory Response}$$

Explore the Cardiac Infection Model

$$(\text{Pathogen} + \text{Host Factors} \xrightarrow{\text{Cardiac Infection}} \text{Inflammatory Response}),$$ delving into the molecular interactions triggering cardiac infections.

Immunomodulation Equation:

$$\text{Immunomodulation} = \frac{\text{Immune Response}}{\text{Pathogen Load}}$$

Peek into the Immunomodulation Equation, showcasing the balance between immune response and pathogen load in the context of cardiac infections.

Embark on a mathematical and molecular journey through Cardiac Infections, enhancing understanding with diverse formulas and equations.

20.6 Cardiac Pathology Case Studies

Embark on a dynamic exploration of Cardiac Pathology Case Studies, unraveling intricate details through mathematical formulas and chemical equations.

Cardiac Risk Score (CRS):

$$CRS = \frac{\text{Cardiac Biomarkers} + \text{Age Factor} - \text{Physical Activity Factor}}{\text{Dietary Factor} \times \text{Stress Level}}$$

Dive into the Cardiac Risk Score (CRS), a comprehensive metric assessing cardiac health, combining cardiac biomarkers, age, physical activity, dietary habits, and stress level.

Cardiac Pathology Model:

$$\text{Genetics} + \text{Environmental Factors} \xrightarrow{\text{Cardiac Pathology}} \text{Functional Abnormalities}$$

Explore the Cardiac Pathology Model (Genetics + Environmental Factors $\xrightarrow{\text{Cardiac Pathology}}$ Functional Abnormalities), unraveling the molecular intricacies contributing to cardiac disorders.

Cardiac Rehabilitation Progress Equation:

$$\text{Rehabilitation Progress} = \frac{\text{Exercise Intensity} \times \text{Dietary Adherence}}{\text{Stress Management}}$$

Peek into the Cardiac Rehabilitation Progress Equation, a guide to monitoring recovery, factoring in exercise intensity, dietary adherence, and stress management.

Embark on a mathematical and molecular journey through Cardiac Pathology Case Studies, enhancing understanding with diverse formulas and equations.

www.ingramcontent.com/pod-product-compliance
Lightning Source LLC
Chambersburg PA
CBHW082337270726
48658CB00017B/2882